Diabetic Desserts for Beginners + Diet

Easy Low Sugar Recipes for Losing Weight and Healthy Living, Great for Beginners + Complete Guide on How to Lose Weight With Simple Recipes With Low Carbohydrates

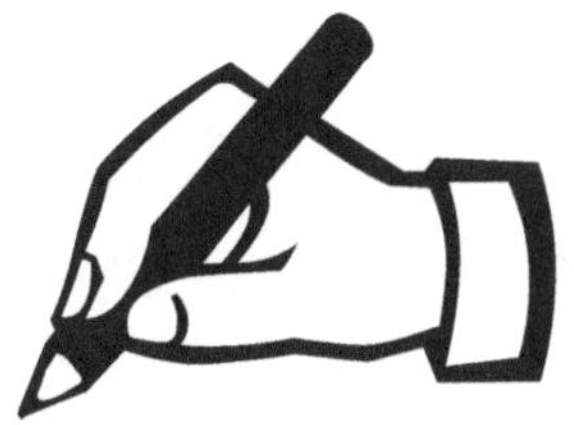

By

Felicity Bath

CONTENTS

DIABETIC DIET

STEWS, CHILIES AND CURRIES

STIR-FRIES

MEATS

CASSEROLES

"BREADED" FRIED FOOD

PIZZA

SIDE DISHES

CROCKPOT

FISH

SWEET

Introduction

Congratulations on purchasing your copy of *Diabetic Desserts for Beginners,* and thank you for doing so. This cookbook will guide you to ways of enjoying diabetic desserts for beginners or pros, and it will help you prepare sugar-free or low-sugar desserts with simple and easy-to-find ingredients.

If you have prediabetes or diabetes, your physician will probably suggest you meet with a professional to create a balanced meal plan. You need to keep your blood sugar at an acceptable level. Doing so helps prevent high blood pressure, helps eliminate heart disease risk, and keeps your weight in line with your frame and activity levels.

As you consume extra fat and calories, your body will respond with a rise in your blood glucose. Always follow a diabetes diet, which is based on eating three, regularly scheduled meals daily.

Suggested Foods

Dietary fiber moderates how your body digests the food you eat and helps control blood sugar levels. Choose healthy carbohydrates and foods containing fiber, including:

- Low-fat dairy products (cheese & milk)
- Legumes (peas & beans)
- Whole grains
- Fruits
- Vegetables
- Nuts
- Whole grains

Two times each week, prepare a delicious platter of fish to provide essential omega-3 fatty acids. *Avoid* the king mackerel since it has high levels of mercury. Incorporate a serving of sardines for a snack or a piece of salmon for dinner.

Foods containing polyunsaturated and monounsaturated fats *can* help lower cholesterol levels. Enjoy a few nuts, olives, and avocados. Using oils derived from olives, nuts, peanuts, or canola are good options.

Foods to Avoid

Consider these categories:

- *Cholesterol* is definitely an enemy on the top spot from elements included in animal proteins and high-fat dairy (organ meats, such as liver or egg yolks). Set your goals by not exceeding more than 200 milligrams (mg) daily.
- *Trans fats* include processed baked goods, snacks, stick margarine, and shortening.
- *Saturated fats* include high-fat dairy and animal products, proteins (sausage, bacon, hot dogs, beef & butter). Consume less palm kernel and coconut oils.

- ☐ *Sodium.* Consume under 2,300 mg daily. Add the elements of high blood pressure, and you will further need to lower your intakes.

Each of the recipes has a breakdown of its nutritional values.

Chapter 1

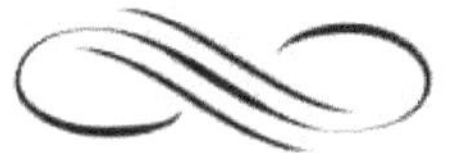

Yogurt Parfait Specialties

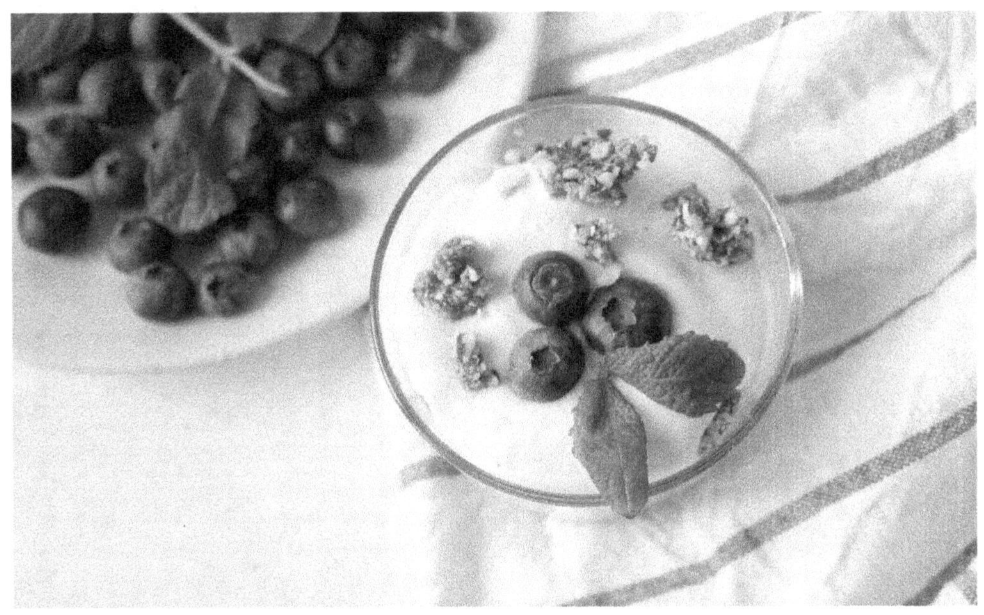

Note; most of the recipes are coded with their diabetic exchanges (DE) when available!

Servings Provided: 4

Time Required: 20 minutes

Macro Counts - Each Serving:

- ☐ Calories: 129
- ☐ Carbs: 27 g
- ☐ Sugar: 17.5 g
- ☐ Fiber: 3.7 g
- ☐ Chol: -0- mg

- ☐ Prot.: 6.4 g
- ☐ Sodium: 75.3 mg
- ☐ Fat Content: 0.4 g (Saturated: -0- g)
  D.E.:
- ☐ Starch: 1
- ☐ Fat: ½
- ☐ Milk: ½

Ingredients Needed:

- ☐ Greek yogurt - fat-free - plain (1 cup)
- ☐ Vanilla (1 tsp.)
- ☐ Honey (2 tbsp.)
- ☐ Fresh raspberries (.5 cup)
- ☐ Lemon peel (.5 tsp.)
- ☐ Fresh blackberries (.5 cup)
- ☐ Fresh blueberries (.5 cup)
- ☐ Multigrain oats & honey cereal (1 cup)
- ☐ Optional Garnish: Lemon peel strips (4 pinches)

Preparation Technique:

1. Finely shred the lemon peel and slice the blackberries.
2. Combine the yogurt with the honey, vanilla, and shredded lemon peel (½ tsp.).
3. Scoop half of the yogurt mixture into four parfait dishes.
4. Garnish the parfait with ½ of the cereal and berries. Repeat the layers.
5. Serve it promptly or cover and chill up to ½ hour. Garnish with lemon peel strips.

Servings Provided: 3.5 dozen

Time Required: 20 minutes + freeze time

Macro Counts - Each Serving:

- ☐ Calories: 75
- ☐ Sodium: 107 mg
- ☐ Carbs: 12 g
- ☐ Sugar: 6 g
- ☐ Fiber: 1 g
- ☐ Prot.: 1 g
- ☐ Chol: -0- mg
- ☐ Fat Content: 2 g (Saturated: 1 g)
  D.E:
- ☐ Starch: 1
- ☐ Fat: ½

Ingredients Needed:

- ☐ Cold milk - fat-free (1.5 cups)
- ☐ Instant chocolate - Sugar-free pudding mix (1.4 oz. pkg.)
- ☐ Frozen & thawed reduced-fat whipped topping (8 oz. carton)
- ☐ Miniature marshmallows (1 cup)
- ☐ Chocolate wafers (9 oz. pkg. - 2 each)

Preparation Technique:

1. Make the filling by whisking the milk and pudding mix for two minutes. Wait for two minutes and mix in the whipped topping, and lastly, the marshmallows.
2. Spread about two tablespoons of the prepared filling onto the bottom of a wafer (for each sandwich). Add another wafer. Stack the sandwiches in covered containers.
3. Freeze until firm (3 hrs.).
4. Remove the container from the freezer. Thaw it and wait for five minutes before serving.

Servings Provided: 2

Time Required: 10 minutes

Macro Counts - Each Serving:

- Calories: 160
- Carbs: 22 g
- Fiber: 3 g
- Sugar: 18 g
- Chol: -0- mg
- Fat Content: 5 g (Sat.: -0- g)
- Protein: 10 g
- Sodium: 33 mg
  D.E:
- Starch: 1
- Fat: 1
- Fruit: ½

Ingredients Needed:

- Halved fresh strawberries (.25 cup)
- Fresh raspberries, blueberries & blackberries (.25 cup each)
- Honey - divided (3 tsp.)
- F.F. Greek yogurt - plain (.5 cup)
- Pomegranate juice (2 tbsp.)
- Chopped walnuts - toasted (2 tbsp.)

Preparation Technique:

1. Toss the berries and one teaspoon of honey. Spoon the berries into two dessert dishes.
2. Combine the pomegranate juice with the yogurt and remaining honey. Scoop it over the berries. Sprinkle with walnuts and serve.

Servings Provided: 4

Time Required: 20 minutes + chill time

Macro Counts - Each Serving:

- With ¼ cup of sauce:
- Calories: 166
- Carbs: 16 g
- Sugar: 11 g
- Fiber: 4 g
- Chol: 132 mg
- Fat Content: 9 g (Saturated: 5 g)
- Protein: 4 g
- Sodium: 34 mg
  D.E:
- Starch: ½
- Fat: 1 ½
- Fruit: ½

Ingredients Needed:

- Half-&-Half cream (1 cup)
- Egg yolks (2 large)
- Sugar (2 tbsp.)
- Vanilla extract (2 tsp.)
- Fresh berries (2 cups)

Preparation Technique:

1. Use a small heavy saucepan to mix the cream with the egg yolks and sugar. Simmer using the low-temperature setting until the mixture is 'just' thickened and reads at least 160° F/71° C on a thermometer. *Don't boil.*
2. Put the mixture into a mixing container and mix in the vanilla. Pop it into the fridge, covered until it's cold. Serve over fresh berries.

Chapter 2

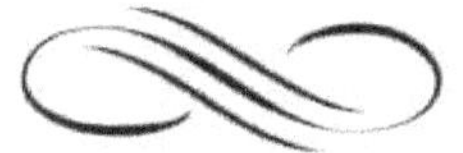

Smoothies & Frozen Treats

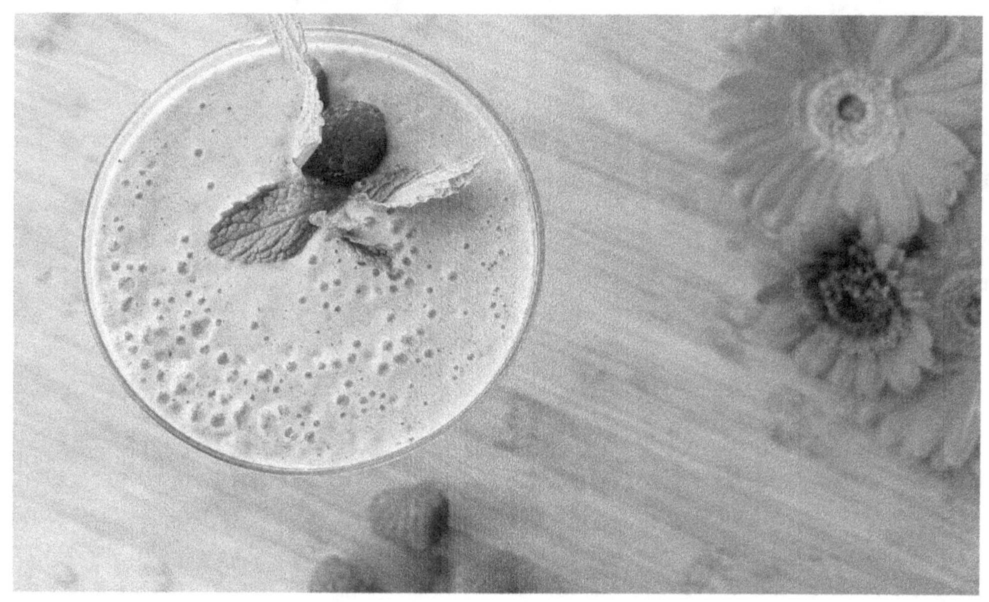

Enjoy a delicious smoothie for breakfast or dessert!

Smoothies

Servings Provided: 2

Time Required: 5 minutes

Macro Counts - Each Serving:

- ☐ Calories: 319
- ☐ Carbs: 12.1 g
- ☐ Fiber: 5.5g
- ☐ Sugar: 2.4 g
- ☐ Chol: -0- mg
- ☐ Protein: 2.3 g

- ☐ Sodium: 180.2 mg
- ☐ Fat Content: 30.6 g (Saturated: 23.4 g)
- ☐ Net Carbs: 6.6 g

Ingredients Needed:

- ☐ Ripe avocado (half of 1)
- ☐ Cocoa powder (3 tbsp.)
- ☐ Coconut milk - full-fat (1 cup)
- ☐ Water (.5 cup/1.2 dl)
- ☐ Lime juice (1 tsp.)
- ☐ Mineral salt (1 pinch)
- ☐ Liquid Stevia (6-7 drops)
- ☐ To Garnish: Fresh mint (as desired)

Preparation Technique:

1. Add all of the ingredients into the blender.
2. Mix using the high-speed setting until it's mixed and creamy. If desired, add more liquid stevia to taste.
3. Top it off using a sprig of fresh mint and serve.

Servings Provided: 2

Time Required: 5 minutes

Macro Counts - Each Serving:

- ☐ Calories: 166
- ☐ Carbs: 4.1 g
- ☐ Sugar: 1.2 g
- ☐ Fiber: 3.3 g
- ☐ Chol: -0- mg
- ☐ Prot.: 17.6 g
- ☐ Sodium: 49.1 mg
- ☐ Fat Content: 9.2 g (Saturated: 6 g)

- ☐ Net Carbs: 0.8 g

Ingredients Needed:

- ☐ Unsweetened almond milk (.5 cup/125 ml)
- ☐ Chopped strawberries (2 oz./50 g)
- ☐ Crushed ice (3 cups/750 ml)
- ☐ Pea/vanilla protein powder (.33 cup/40 g)
- ☐ Psyllium husk powder (.5 tsp.)
- ☐ Coconut oil (1 tbsp.)
- ☐ Liquid Stevia (5 – 10 drops)

Preparation Technique:

1. Put the ice cubes in a blender and allow them to sit for five minutes. You want them to melt slightly, so the blender has some traction.
2. Add the rest of the fixings and mix until it's light pink and creamy.
3. Pour it into a serving bowl and top it off using desired toppings.

Servings Provided: 1

Time Required: 5 minutes

Macro Counts - Each Serving:

- ☐ Calories: 309
- ☐ Carbs: 35.2 g
- ☐ Fiber: 14.8 g
- ☐ Protein: 18.4 g
- ☐ Fat Content: 11.2 g

Ingredients Needed:

- ☐ Almond milk - unsweetened (1 cup)
- ☐ Unsweetened - plain yogurt/plain kefir (.5 cup)
- ☐ Stevia - ex. Sweet Leaf brand (2 packets)
- ☐ Unsweetened cocoa powder (1 tbsp.)

- [ ] English Toffee stevia (5 drops)
- [ ] Creamy peanut/almond butter & no sugar added (1 heaping tbsp.)
- [ ] PaleoFiber powder/chia seed/ground flaxseed meal (1 tbsp.)
- [ ] Collagen hydrolysate/Vanilla protein powder of your choice (1 tbsp.)
- [ ] Vanilla extract (.5 tsp.)

Preparation Technique:

1. Toss the fixings into your blender.
2. Set using the high setting, pulsing until thoroughly combined.

Servings Provided: 3 medium

Time Required: 12 minutes

Macro Counts - Each Serving:

- [ ] Calories: 123
- [ ] Carbs: 31 g
- [ ] Sugar: 17 g
- [ ] Fiber: 5 g
- [ ] Prot.: 2 g
- [ ] Sodium: 30 mg

Ingredients Needed:

- [ ] Water (1.5 cups/375g)
- [ ] Fresh kale or spinach (2 cups/134g)
- [ ] Fresh mint (.5 cup/22.5g)
- [ ] Ripe green pear (1)
- [ ] Chilled green or Moscato grapes (20)
- [ ] Ripe green apple (1)
- [ ] Ice cubes (12)
- [ ] Cinnamon (.75 tsp)
- [ ] Stevia (1 tsp.) or Agave nectar (1 tbsp./ as desired)
- [ ] Lime (1 - juiced, or more to taste)

☐ Note: Use organic produce if available

Preparation Technique:

1. Remove the core from the apples and pear and chop them into chunks. Roughly chop the kale/spinach and mint.
2. Pour the cold water into the blender with a small handful of the apple and pear chunks. Blend till the mixture is thoroughly liquified. Continue adding them until they are gone.
3. Add the greens and mint the same way. Blend in batches if needed until all of the greens have been incorporated. Add the grapes, ice cubes, agave/stevia, cinnamon, and lime juice.
4. Blend the mixture until the ice cubes are thoroughly crushed, and the mixture is smooth (1 min.).
5. Serve for an energized day!
6. Note: Please be sure to follow the steps in the order suggested. Otherwise, they won't blend properly.

Servings Provided: 1

Time Required: 5 minutes

Macro Counts - Each Serving:

☐ Calories: 167
☐ Carbs: 11 g
☐ Sugar: 6 g
☐ Fiber: 2 g
☐ Chol: 8 mg
☐ Prot.: 16 g
☐ Sodium: 161 mg
☐ Fat Content: 6 g (Saturated: 1 g)

Ingredients Needed:

☐ Strawberries (5 medium)
☐ Unsweetened almond/soy milk (1 cup)

- ☐ Greek-style yogurt - L.F. (.5 cup)
- ☐ Ice (6 cubes)

Preparation Technique:

1. Toss each of the ingredients into a blender, mixing until creamy.
2. Serve in a chilled glass with a fresh strawberry!

Servings Provided: 1

Time Required: 5 minutes

Macro Counts - Each Serving:

- ☐ Calories: 276
- ☐ Fiber: 14.3 g
- ☐ Carbs: 44.7 g
- ☐ Prot.: 16.7 g
- ☐ Sodium: mg
- ☐ Fat Content: 2.6 g

Ingredients Needed:

- ☐ Almond milk - unsweetened (1 cup)
- ☐ Unsweetened plain yogurt/unsweetened plain kefir (.5 cup)
- ☐ Stevia (2 packets)
- ☐ Banana (¼ of 1 small)
- ☐ Fresh or frozen strawberries (.5 cup)
- ☐ Paleo Fiber powder/ground flaxseed meal/chia seed (1 tbsp.)
- ☐ Collagen hydrolysate/vanilla protein powder of your choice (1 tbsp.)
- ☐ Vanilla extract (.5 tsp.)

Preparation Technique:

1. Toss all of the fixings into a blender.
2. Mix using the high-speed setting.

Servings Provided: 1

Time Required: 5 minutes

Macro Counts - Each Serving:

- Calories: 255
- Carbs: 39 g
- Sugar: 24 g
- Fiber: 7.8 g
- Protein: 5.6 g
- Sodium: 168.4 mg
- Fat Content: 11.1 g (Saturated: 1.1 g)
  D.E.:
- Fat: 2
- Fruit: 2 ½

Ingredients Needed:

- Frozen strawberries (1 cup)
- Freshly chopped pineapple (1 cup)
- Chilled unsweetened almond milk (.75 cup + more if needed)
- Almond butter (1 tbsp.)

Preparation Technique:

1. Toss the pineapple, strawberries, almond butter, and almond milk into a blender.
2. Pulse until it's creamy smooth, adding more almond milk, if needed, for desired consistency.
3. Serve promptly.

Other Unique Frozen Treats

When you prepare ice pops, you can use molds such as the ones provided by Tupperware or use a paper cup. Cover the cup with a piece of aluminum foil. Poke a wooden stick/handle in through the foil and freeze the pop.

Some of the recipes will suggest using an ice cream maker. In its place, use a shallow metal pan or ice cube trays to freeze the pops. Pop it in the freezer until firm (6 hrs.). Once it is frozen, use a mallet to break it apart. Pop it into the food processor to mix until creamy smooth.

Servings Provided: 10

Time Required: 10 minutes + freeze time

Macro Counts - Each Serving:

- Calories: 51
- Carbs: 8 g
- Sugar: 6 g
- Fiber: 2 g
- Chol: 4 mg
- Prot.: 2 g
- Sodium: 19 mg
- Fat Content: 2 g (Saturated: 1 g)
  D.E.:
- Starch: ½

Ingredients Needed:

- Whole milk - divided (1.75 cups)
- Honey (1-2 tbsp.)
- Vanilla extract (.25 tsp.)
- Blueberries - fresh (1 cup)
- Raspberries - fresh (1.5 cups)
- Paper cups or freezer pop molds & sticks (10 @ about 6 tbsp. each)

Preparation Technique:

1. Pour the water into a safe container and warm ¼ cup of milk in the microwave. Stir in the honey and rest of the milk (1.5 cups), and vanilla.
2. Portion the berries into the molds, and pour milk into the mixture. Place the tops onto the molds with holders.
3. Pop them in the freezer until they are solid to serve.

Servings Provided: 1

Time Required: 2 hours

Macro Counts - Each Serving:

- Calories: 127
- Carbs: 8.1 g
- Sugar: 4.4 g
- Chol: 9.7 mg
- Protein: 20.1 g
- Sodium: 150 mg
- Fat Content: 2.2 g (Saturated: 0.4 g)
- Net Carbs: 5.6 g

Ingredients Needed:

- Almond milk - unsweetened (.5 cup or 120 ml)
- Fat-free Greek yogurt (2.5 oz./75 g)
- Vanilla protein powder (.5 oz./15 g)
- Unsweetened cocoa powder (1 tsp.)
- Stevia (2 tbsp./to taste)
- Vanilla extract (1 tsp.)
- Optional: Almonds & berries
- Useful: Blender/whisk

Preparation Technique:

1. Blend the yogurt with the protein powder, stevia, cocoa, and almond milk. Place the mixture in your freezer or ice cream machine.

2. If making in the freezer, remove the ice cream out after an hour and gently stir using a spoon to avoid a large ice block. Repeat every ½ hour until the ice cream has the right consistency (2 hours total).

3. After the waiting time has elapsed, take the ice cream from the freezer five to ten minutes before you are prepared to serve it.

Servings Provided: 3 cups

Time Required: 15 minutes + freeze time

Macro Counts - Each Serving:

- ½ cup per portion:
- Calories: 181
- Carbs: 29 g
- Sugar: 16 g
- Fiber: 4 g
- Chol: -0- mg
- Prot.: 3 g
- Fat Content: 7 g (Saturated: 2 g)
- Sodium: 35 mg
  D.E:
- Starch: ½
- Fat: 1
- Fruit: 1

Ingredients Needed:

- Bananas - peeled & frozen (5 medium)
- Unsweetened coconut - finely shredded (2 tbsp.)
- Almond milk (.33 cup)
- Vanilla extract (1 tsp.)
- Creamy peanut butter (2 tbsp.)
- Chopped walnuts (.25 cup)
- Raisins (3 tbsp.)

Preparation Technique:

1. Place the bananas, peanut butter, milk, vanilla, and coconut in a food processor. Close the lid and blend the mixture.
2. Pour it into a freezer container, and fold in the walnuts and raisins. Freeze for two to four hours before serving.

Servings Provided: 10 pops

Time Required: 15 minutes + freeze time

Macro Counts - Each Serving:

- ☐ Calories: 60
- ☐ Carbs: 9 g
- ☐ Sugar: 8 g
- ☐ Fiber: 1 g
- ☐ Chol: -0- mg
- ☐ Prot.: 6 g
- ☐ Fat Content: -0-g
- ☐ Sodium: 28 mg
- ☐ **D.E:**
- ☐ Starch: 1

Ingredients Needed:

- ☐ Plastic or paper cups (10 @ 3 oz. each)
- ☐ Honey Greek yogurt - fat-free (2.75 cups)
- ☐ Fresh berries - mixed (1 cup)
- ☐ Water (.25 cup)
- ☐ Sugar (2 tbsp.)
- ☐ Wooden pop sticks (10)

Preparation Technique:

1. Fill each cup with yogurt (¼ cup).
2. Prepare the food processor. Toss in the berries, water, and sugar. Swirl it until the berries are thoroughly chopped.
3. Scoop 1.5 tablespoons of the berry mixture into each cup. Gently stir using a popsicle stick to swirl.

Top each of the cups with foil and add the pop sticks in through foil. Freeze until firm.

Grab any time for a delicious treat!

Servings Provided: 1 dozen

Time Required: 15 minutes + freeze time

Macro Counts - Each Serving:

- Calories: 60
- Carbs: 13 g
- Sugar: 10 g
- Fiber: 1 g
- Chol: 2 mg
- Prot.: 2 g
- Sodium: 23 mg
- Fat Content: 1 g (Saturated: -0- g)
  D.E:
- Starch: 1

Ingredients Needed:

- Raspberry yogurt (2.25 cups)
- Lemon juice (2 tbsp.)
- Ripe bananas (2 medium)
- Freezer pop mold/paper cups (12 @ 3 oz. each) and wooden pop sticks

Preparation Technique:

1. Cut the banana into chunks.
2. Scoop the yogurt, lemon juice, and bananas into a blender. Put the top on the blender and mix until it's creamy.
3. Scoop the prepared mixture into the cups and add the holders. Freeze until they are firm.

Servings Provided: 8

Time Required: 10 minutes + freeze time

Macro Counts - Each Serving:

- Calories: 94
- Carbs: 11 g
- Sugar: 10 g
- Sodium: 33 mg
- Fiber: -0- g
- Chol: -0- mg
- Fat Content: 4 g (Saturated: 1 g)
- Protein: 4 g
  D.E:
- Starch: 1
- Fat: ½

Ingredients Needed:

- Soy milk - vanilla (1 cup)
- Fat-free milk (.5 cup)
- Vanilla Greek yogurt - fat-free (.75 cup)
- Nutella (1/3 cup)
- Paper cups/pop molds (8 @ 3 ounces each) & wooden pop sticks

Preparation Technique:

1. Pour the milk, yogurt, and Nutella into a blender.
2. Securely close the top and mix until it's creamy. Scoop it into the holders and seal the tops with foil, adding the sticks.
3. Freeze until firm.

Servings Provided: 6

Time Required: 15 minutes + freeze time

Macro Counts - Each Serving:

- Calories: 31
- Carbs: 8 g
- Fiber: 1 g
- Sugar: 6 g
- Chol: -0- mg
- Sodium: -0- mg
- Fat Content: -0- g (Saturated: -0- g)
- Prot.: -0- g
  D.E:
- Fruit: ½

Ingredients Needed:

- Orange juice (.25 cup)
- Grated lemon zest (1 tsp.)
- Sugar (4 tsp.)
- Lemon juice (.25 cup)
- Fresh apricots (1 cup/4-5 medium)
- Ice cubes (.5 cup)
  ****
- Optional: 1 teaspoon minced fresh mint (1 tsp.)
- Molds & sticks for the pops (6 @ 6 tbsp. each)

Preparation Technique:

1. Slice the apricots and make the juice and zest from the lemon.
2. Toss the first six fixings into a blender (up to the line**); cover and process until blended. Add in freshly minced mint.
3. Pour the mixture into molds and freeze until firm.

Servings Provided: 12

Time Required: 15 minutes + freeze time

Macro Counts - Each Serving:

- ☐ Calories: 55
- ☐ Carbs: 11 g
- ☐ Sugar: 10 g
- ☐ Chol: 2 mg
- ☐ Fiber: 1 g
- ☐ Prot.: 2 g
- ☐ Fat Content: 1 g (Saturated: -0- g)
- ☐ Sodium: 24 mg
  D.E:
- ☐ Starch: 1

Ingredients Needed:

- ☐ Vanilla yogurt - divided (1.75 cups)
- ☐ Honey - divided (2 tbsp.)
- ☐ Fresh strawberries - sliced & divided (1.25 cups)
- ☐ Frozen or fresh blueberries - thawed & divided (1.25 cups)
- ☐ Freezer popsicle molds/paper cups (12 @ 3 oz. each) & wooden pop sticks

Preparation Technique:

1. Measure and add one tablespoon honey, two tablespoons yogurt, and one cup strawberries in a blender. Place the lid on tightly and process until blended. Pour it into a small, holding container.
2. Chop the rest of the strawberries and add them to the mixture.
3. Use a blender to process the rest of the honey with two tablespoons of yogurt and one cup of blueberries. Transfer them to another container. Fold in the rest of the blueberries.
4. Prepare the molds. Scoop the strawberry mixture (1 tbsp.), yogurt (2 tbsp.), and blueberry mixture (1 tbsp.).
5. Top with the popsicle sticks or cover the cups with a layer of foil. Freeze until firm.

Servings Provided: 8

Time Required: 4 hours 45 minutes

Macro Counts - Each Serving:

- Calories: 94
- Carbs: 24g
- Fiber: 1.1 g
- Sugar: 22.6 g
- Chol: -0- mg
- Prot.: 0.7 g
- Sodium: 3.3 mg
- Fat Content: 0.2 g (Saturated: -0- g)
  D.E.:
- Fruit: ½
- Other Carbohydrate: 1 ½

Ingredients Needed:

- White grape juice (1 cup)
- Frozen/fresh ripe peaches (about 4/4 cups)
- Lemon juice (1 tbsp.)
- Sugar (.5 cup)
- Also Needed: Ice cream maker**

Preparation Technique:

1. Set up the food processor. Quarter and puree the peaches.
2. Whisk both of the juices and sugar in a saucepan. Warm it using the medium-temperature setting, stirring until it's liquified.
3. Combine and chill the fixings (syrup and fruit puree) in the fridge (4 hs.).
4. Add the sorbet mixture into an ice cream maker.
5. It will be delicious for up to one week. Be sure to slightly soften it before serving.

Servings Provided: 2.5 cups/.5 cup portions

Time Required: 10 minutes + freeze time

Macro Counts - Each Serving:

- Calories: 104
- Carbs: 26 g
- Sugar: 15 g
- Fiber: 2 g
- Chol: 1 mg
- Prot.: 2 g
- Sodium: 15 mg
- Fat Content: 0 g (Saturated: 0 g)
  D.E:
- Fruit: 1
- Starch: ½

Ingredients Needed:

- Ripe bananas (4 medium)
- Fat-free plain yogurt (.5 cup)
- Maple syrup (1-2 tbsp.)
- Frozen unsweetened raspberries (.5 cup)
- Optional: Fresh raspberries

Preparation Technique:

1. Thinly slice the bananas and transfer them into a large plastic zipper-type freezer bag. Arrange the slices in a single layer; freeze overnight.
2. Finely chop the bananas in a food processor.
3. Mix in the yogurt, maple syrup, and raspberries. Pulse the mixture a few times just until smooth, scraping sides as needed.
4. Serve immediately, adding fresh berries as desired.

Servings Provided: 6

Time Required: 5 minutes + chill time of 3 hours

Macro Counts - Each Serving:

- ☐ Calories: 73
- ☐ Carbs: 14.2 g
- ☐ Sugar: 8 g
- ☐ Fiber: 2 g
- ☐ Chol: 1.7 mg
- ☐ Protein: 3.5 g
- ☐ Sodium: 67 mg
- ☐ Fat Content: 0.5 g (Saturated: 0.1 g)
- ☐ Net Carbs: 12.2 g

Ingredients Needed:

- ☐ Old-fashioned oats (.25 cup/22 g)
- ☐ Low fat cottage cheese (4 oz./115 g)
- ☐ Strawberries (1.5 lb./680 g)
- ☐ Lemon juice (4 oz./about 4 lemons/115 g)
- ☐ Liquid Stevia (5 drops)
- ☐ Essential: Food processor or high-powered blender

Preparation Technique:

1. Pulse the oats until they're powdery.
2. Add the cottage cheese, strawberries, stevia, and lemon juice.
3. Pulse the mixture until smooth. Don't add any liquid!
4. Prepare the six molds and freeze until firm (3 hrs.).

Servings Provided: 8

Time Required: 25 minutes + cool time

Macro Counts - Each Serving:

- ☐ Calories: 72
- ☐ Carbs: 16 g
- ☐ Fiber: 1 g
- ☐ Sugar: 14 g
- ☐ Sodium: 18 mg
- ☐ Prot.: 2 g
- ☐ Chol: 2 mg
- ☐ Fat Content: -0- g (Saturated: -0- g)
  D.E:
- ☐ Starch: 1

Ingredients Needed:

- ☐ Chopped fresh or frozen rhubarb (3 cups)
- ☐ Sugar (.25 cup)
- ☐ Water (3 tbsp.)
- ☐ Strawberry yogurt (1 cup)
- ☐ Unsweetened applesauce (.5 cup)
- ☐ Finely chopped fresh strawberries (.25 cup)
- ☐ Optional: Red food coloring(2 drops)
- ☐ Paper cups/freezer pop molds (8 @ 3 ounces each) and wooden sticks

Preparation Technique:

1. Slice the rhubarb into ½-inch cuts and mix with the water and sugar in a big saucepan. Once boiling, reduce the temperature setting to simmer, uncovered, until thick and blended (10-15 min.). Remove 3/4 cup mixture to a bowl; cool completely. (Save remaining rhubarb for another use.)
2. Add the yogurt, applesauce, and strawberries to the bowl; stir until blended. If desired, tint with food coloring.

3. Fill each mold or cup with about 1/4 cup of the rhubarb mixture.

4. Top the molds with holders and top cups with a layer of foil. Push the sticks through the foil. Freeze until they are firm.

Servings Provided: 8

Time Required: 20 minutes + freeze time

Macro Counts - Each Serving:

- ☐ Calories: 153
- ☐ Carbs: 27 g
- ☐ Sugar: 18 g
- ☐ Fiber: 2 g
- ☐ Chol: 1 mg
- ☐ Prot.: 1 g
- ☐ Fat Content: 3 g (Saturated: 3 g)
- ☐ Sodium: 163 mg
  D.E:
- ☐ Starch: 2
- ☐ Fat: ½

Ingredients Needed:

- ☐ Strawberry sorbet (2 cups)
- ☐ Cold milk- fat-free (1 cup)
- ☐ Instant vanilla pudding mix - sugar-free (1 oz. pkg.)
- ☐ Reduced-fat whipped topping (frozen 8 oz. carton)
- ☐ Sliced fresh strawberries
- ☐ Also Suggested: 8x4-inch loaf pan

Preparation Technique:

1. Thaw the whipped topping.
2. Line the loaf pan with plastic wrap. Slightly soften the sorbet and add it to the pan. Freeze it for about 15 minutes.
3. Meanwhile, whisk the pudding mix with the milk for two minutes. It will be soft-set soon (2 min.). Mix and add the thawed topping over the sorbet. Cover the container to freeze and set for four hours to overnight.

4. Transfer the pan to the countertop to slightly thaw before serving (10-15 min.). Flip and invert the dessert onto a plate. Discard the plastic and slice the sorbet. Lastly, slice the strawberries and sprinkle them over the top to serve.

Chapter 3

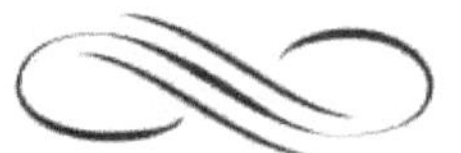

Muffins

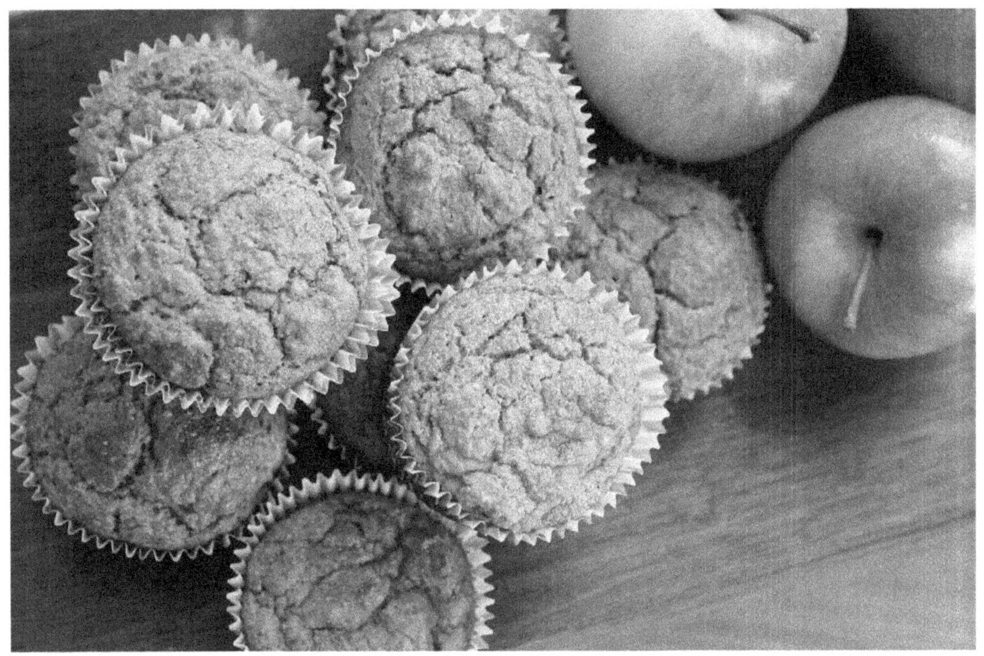

Servings Provided: 6

Time Required: 30-35 minutes

Macro Counts - Each Serving:

- ☐ Calories: 270
- ☐ Carbs: 34 g
- ☐ Sugar: 17 g
- ☐ Fiber: 3 g
- ☐ Chol: 30 mg
- ☐ Prot.: 5 g
- ☐ Sodium: 360 mg

☐ Fat Content: 14 g (Saturated: 1.4 g)

Ingredients Needed:

☐ Bak. powder (1 tsp.)

☐ Flour - whole wheat (1 cup)

☐ Cinnamon - ground (1 tsp.)

☐ Bak. soda (.25 tsp.)

☐ Kosher salt (.5 tsp.)

****

☐ Canola oil (.25 cup)

☐ Brown sugar (.33 cup)

☐ Egg (1 large)

☐ Vanilla sugar-free yogurt (.33 cup)

☐ Carrot (.75 cup)

☐ Banana (.5 cup)

☐ Vanilla extract (1 tsp.)

☐ Pecans (.25 cup)

Preparation Technique:

1. Place paper/foil liners in a six-cup muffin tin.
2. Mash the bananas, shred the carrot, and chop the pecans. Set them aside.
3. Combine the first five fixings (up to the line **) in a large mixing container.
4. Whisk the oil with the sugar and egg in another container. Mix in the yogurt, carrots, banana, and vanilla. Stir the oil mix into the flour mixture in a big mixing container. Fold in the pecans.
5. Scoop the batter evenly into the muffin cups.
6. Set a timer to bake at 375° Fahrenheit or 191° Celsius until muffins are lightly browned as desired (22 min.).

Servings Provided: 8

Time Required: 40 minutes

Macro Counts - Each Serving:

- ☐ Calories: 189
- ☐ Carbs: 17.3 g
- ☐ Sugar: 5.6 g
- ☐ Fiber: 3.9 g
- ☐ Chol: -0- mg
- ☐ Prot.: 3.8 g
- ☐ Sodium: 226.5 mg
- ☐ Fat Content: 13.9 g (Saturated: 8.4 g)

Ingredients Needed:

- ☐ Dry Components:
- ☐ Almond flour (1.75 cups/170 g)
- ☐ Baking soda (1 tsp.)
- ☐ Tapioca starch (.25 cup/.32 g)
- ☐ Granulated sweetener of choice - ex. Xylitol (.5 cup/15 g)
- ☐ Baking powder - gluten-free (1 tsp.)
- ☐ Nutmeg (1 tsp.)
- ☐ Cinnamon (1 tbsp.)
- ☐ Salt (1 tsp.)
- ☐ Cloves (.25 tsp.)
- ☐ Wet Components:
- ☐ Coconut oil (.33 cup/0.8 dl)
- ☐ Vanilla extract (1 tsp.)
- ☐ Banana - overripe and mashed (1 medium)
- ☐ Shredded carrots (1.5 cups/75 g)
- ☐ Flax meal (4 tbsp.) + Water (.5 cup/2.2 dl) = a flax egg for vegan OR
- ☐ *Eggs (2 large) if you are not vegan

Preparation Technique:

1. Set the oven temperature at 350° Fahrenheit or 177 ° Celsius.
2. Prepare a muffin tray with paper cups.
3. Toss each of the dry fixings into a mixing container. Thoroughly whisk to remove all of the lumps.
4. Whisk ½ cup of water with the flax meal until it becomes a "flax egg." Wait for five minutes.
5. Use your thumb to make a hole in the middle of the dry components. Mix in the flax egg, coconut oil, and vanilla extract. Combine to create a rough dough, but avoid over-mixing.
6. Mash the bananas and shred the carrots. Toss them into the mixture until just incorporated.
7. Scoop the muffin batter into the cups filling them to the tops.
8. Bake the muffins for 35 to 40 minutes.
9. Cool in the tray for ten minutes. At that time, transfer them to a rack to cool slightly before serving.

Servings Provided: 12

Time Required: 1 hour

Macro Counts - Each Serving:

- ☐ Calories: 217
- ☐ Carbs: 14.2g
- ☐ Fiber: 4.6g
- ☐ Sugar: 2.5 g
- ☐ Chol: 62 mg
- ☐ Prot.: 4.9 g
- ☐ Fat Content: 14.1 g (Saturated: 9.1 g)
- ☐ Sodium: 125.4 mg
- ☐ Net Carbs: 9.6 g

Ingredients Needed:

- ☐ Canned pumpkin puree (1 cup)
- ☐ Coconut flour (.5 cup)
- ☐ Blanched almond flour (.75 cup)
- ☐ Tapioca or arrowroot starch (3 tbsp.)
- ☐ Baking powder (1 tbsp.)
- ☐ Stevia (.5 cup)
- ☐ Salt (.25 tsp.)
- ☐ Nutmeg (1 pinch)
- ☐ Cinnamon (1 tbsp.)
- ☐ Egg whites (4/.5 cup)
- ☐ Egg yolks (4)
- ☐ Coconut oil (melted @ .5 cup)
- ☐ Vanilla extract (1.5 tsp.)
- ☐ Frozen raspberries (1.5 cups)
- ☐ Liquid stevia (10 drops)
- ☐ Needed: 12-count muffin tin

Preparation Technique:

1. Prep the oven temperature to reach 350° Fahrenheit or 177 ° Celsius.
2. Place paper liners in the muffin cups.
3. Sift or whisk the coconut flour with the almond flour, stevia, tapioca starch, baking powder, nutmeg, cinnamon, and sea salt.
4. Whisk and mix in the egg yolks, pumpkin puree, vanilla, stevia drops, and coconut oil.
5. Use another container and briskly whisk the egg whites to create stiff white peaks. Mix in the frozen raspberries and add them into the muffin batter using a spoon or spatula.
6. Scoop the batter into the cups, filling them to the top of the muffin papers.
7. Set the timer to bake for 25 minutes. Cool in the muffin tray for five minutes. At that time, arrange them on a cooling rack until ready to serve.

Chapter 4

Custard - Pudding and Mousse

Servings Provided: 1

Time Required: 5 minutes

Macro Counts - Each Serving:

- Calories: 122
- Carbs: 19.5 g
- Sugar: 9.3 g
- Fiber: 5.3 g
- Chol: -0- mg
- Prot.: 11.3 g
- Sodium: 153.8 mg
- Fat Content: 0.2 g (Saturated: 0.1 g)
- Net Carbs: 14.2

Ingredients Needed:

- Egg whites (2) or Liquid egg white (90 g)
- Stevia (1 tbsp.)
- Frozen banana (2 oz./60 g)
- Frozen raspberry (1.75 oz./45 g)
- Optional: Fresh berries

Preparation Technique:

1. Whisk or blend the egg whites with the stevia until they are firm (1-2 minutes). Mix in the berries and banana.
2. Once it's all pink and smooth, enjoy it in a serving dish with a garnish of fresh berries.

Servings Provided: 4

Time Required: 15 minutes + chill time

Macro Counts - Each Serving:

- ¾ cup serving:
- Calories: 165
- Carbs: 21 g
- Fiber: -0- g
- Sugar: 17 g
- Chol: 97 mg
- Protein: 7 g
- Sodium: 80 mg
- Fat Content: 6 g (Saturated: 4 g)
  D.E:
- Starch: 1
- Reduced-fat Milk: ½

Ingredients Needed:

- Reduced-fat eggnog (2 cups)
- Unflavored gelatin (2 tsp.)
- Ground nutmeg (0.125 tsp. + more to garnish)
- Sugar (2 tbsp.)
- Ground cinnamon (0.125 tsp.)
- Vanilla extract (.5 tsp.)
- Reduced-fat whipped topping - divided (1 cup)

Preparation Technique:

1. Use a small saucepan, and add the gelatin with the eggnog. Warm the pan using the low-temperature setting to liquefy the mixture (1 min.).
2. Mix in the cinnamon, nutmeg, and sugar - stirring until the sugar is liquified. Add the mousse mixture to a small mixing container and combine it with the vanilla. Pop it into the fridge until thickened.

3. Whisk the mixture until it's fluffy. Mix in the whipped topping (¾ cup).

4. Portion the mousse into dessert bowls and pop them into the fridge to set.

5. Garnish with the rest of the whipped topping and a sprinkle of nutmeg to your liking.

Servings Provided: 10

Time Required: 55 minutes + chill time

Macro Counts - Each Serving:

- ☐ Topping Counts Not Included:
- ☐ Calories: 120
- ☐ Carbs: 24 g
- ☐ Sugar: 21 g
- ☐ Fiber: 2 g
- ☐ Chol: 2 mg
- ☐ Protein: 7 g
- ☐ Sodium: 151 mg
- ☐ Fat Content: -0- g (Saturated: -0- g)
  D.E:
- ☐ Starch: 1 ½

Ingredients Needed:

- ☐ Pumpkin (15 oz. can)
- ☐ Egg whites (8 large)
- ☐ Evaporated milk - fat-free (12 oz. can)
- ☐ Milk - fat-free (.5 cup)
- ☐ ************
- ☐ Ground nutmeg (.25 tsp.)
- ☐ Sugar (.75 cup)
- ☐ Ground cloves (.25 tsp.)
- ☐ Cinnamon (1 tsp.)
- ☐ Salt (.25 tsp.)
- ☐ Ground ginger (.5 tsp.)
- ☐ Optional: Sweetened whipped cream + more cinnamon
- ☐ Also Needed:
- ☐ 15x10x1-inch baking pan
- ☐ Ramekins/custard cups (10 @ 6 oz. each)

Preparation Technique:

1. Warm the oven to reach 350° Fahrenheit/177 ° Celsius.
2. Lightly spritz the baking pan with a cooking oil spray.
3. Arrange the ramekins in the baking tray.
4. Whisk the first four fixings (up to the **line) until smooth. Mix in the salt with the spices and sugar. Portion the custard into the custard cups.
5. Bake for 40-45 minutes. Place the pan of custard on a rack to cool.
6. Pop them into the fridge or serve within two hours.
7. Garnish the custard using a portion of whipped cream and a dusting of cinnamon.

Chapter 5

Delicious Cakes

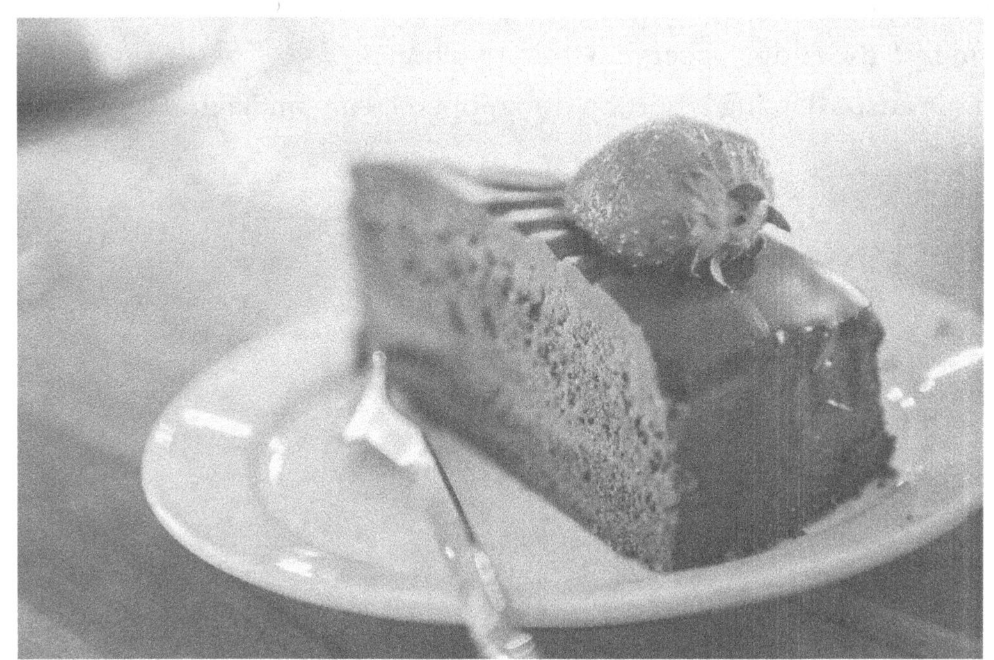

Servings Provided: 10

Time Required: 1 hour 5 minutes

Macro Counts - Each Serving:

- ☐ Calories: 138
- ☐ Carbs: 6.5 g
- ☐ Sugar: 1.8 g
- ☐ Fiber: 1.4 g
- ☐ Chol: 55.5 mg
- ☐ Protein: 3.9 g
- ☐ Sodium: mg

- [ ] Fat Content: 11.5 g (Saturated: 4.3 g)

Ingredients Needed:

- [ ] Ripe banana (.5 cup/2 small)
- [ ] Eggs (3 large)
- [ ] Coconut oil (3 tbsp.)
- [ ] Almond flour (1.5 cups)
- [ ] Xanthan gum (2 tbsp.)
- [ ] Granulated stevia (.33 cup)
- [ ] Baking powder (1.5 tsp.)
- [ ] Cinnamon (2 tsp.)
- [ ] Nutmeg (1 pinch)
- [ ] Pecans or walnuts (.5 cup - crushed)
- [ ] Also Needed: 7.5-inch loaf tin

Preparation Technique:

1. Warm the oven at 350° Fahrenheit/177 ° Celsius.
2. Cover the baking pan using a layer of parchment baking paper. Set aside.
3. Mash the bananas and mix with the eggs and melted coconut oil. Use an electric mixer to thoroughly blend until it's smooth.
4. In another mixing container, combine the almond flour with the xanthan gum, granulated stevia, nutmeg, cinnamon, and baking powder.
5. Combine the dry fixings with the wet and mix until the batter is smooth and incorporated. Fold in the crushed nuts.
6. Empty the prepared batter into the pan. Use a spatula to even the batter.
7. Set a timer to cook for 35 to 40 minutes until done.
8. Remove and cool it for 15 to 20 minutes in the tin.
9. When the loaf is cooled slightly, remove it from the tin and thoroughly cool it before slicing.

Servings Provided: 6

Time Required: 55 minutes

Macro Counts - Each Serving:

- Calories: 168
- Carbs: 21 g
- Sugar: 16 g
- Fiber: 1 g
- Chol: 151 mg
- Protein: 5 g
- Sodium: 83 mg
- Fat Content: 7 g (Saturated: 3 g)
  D.E:
- Starch: 1
- Fat: 1
- Fruit: ½

Ingredients Needed:

- Eggs - separated (4 large)
- Egg white (1 large)
- Butter (2 tbsp.)
- Ripened bananas (1 cup)
- Cornstarch (1 tbsp.)
- Grated lemon zest (.25 tsp.)
- Rum (1 tbsp.)
- Sugar (.33 cup)
- Lemon juice (1 tbsp.)
- Also Needed: 1.5-quart souffle dish

Preparation Technique:

1. Place the egg whites on the countertop for ½ hour. Coat the souffle dish with a spritz of cooking oil spray.

2. Warm a saucepan on the stovetop - set using the medium-temperature setting. Melt the butter. Mash and add the bananas, cornstarch, and sugar, mixing until blended.

3. Wait for it to boil, continually stirring. Cook and stir the mixture for one to two more minutes or until thickened. Empty the mixture into a big mixing container. Mix in the rum, lemon juice, and zest.

4. Fold in a minimal portion of the hot mix into the egg yolks and add all of the fixings back into the bowl, continually mixing. Slightly cool and set aside.

5. In another container, vigorously beat the egg whites to create "stiff" peaks.

6. Slowly mix in ¼ of the egg whites into the banana mixture. Stir in the remainder of the egg whites until combined.

7. Scoop it into the baking dish.

8. Bake at 350° Fahrenheit or 177 ° Celsius until the top is puffed and the center appears set (½ hour). Enjoy it promptly.

Servings Provided: 12

Time Required: 40 minutes + cool time

Macro Counts - Each Serving:

- ☐ Calories: 169
- ☐ Carbs: 25 g
- ☐ Sugar: 10 g
- ☐ Fiber: 1 g
- ☐ Chol: 45 mg
- ☐ Prot.: 4 g
- ☐ Sodium: 261 mg
- ☐ Fat Content: 6 g (Saturated: 4 g)
  D.E:
- ☐ Starch: 1 ½
- ☐ Fat: 1

Ingredients Needed:

- ☐ Unchilled butter (.33 cup)
- ☐ Packed brown sugar (.33 cup)
- ☐ Vanilla extract (2 tsp.)
- ☐ Sugar substitute (equal to 0.75 cup sugar)
- ☐ Unchilled large eggs (2)
- ☐ Water (.5 cup)
- ☐ Baking cocoa (3 tbsp.)
- ☐ Nonfat dry milk powder (.5 cup)
- ☐ Bak. soda (.5 tsp.)
- ☐ A.P. flour (1.33 cups)
- ☐ Salt (.5 tsp.)
- ☐ Bak. powder (1 tsp.)
- ☐ Mashed ripe bananas (1 cup/about 2 medium)
- ☐ Confectioners' sugar
- ☐ Suggested: 9-inch square baking pan

Preparation Technique:

1. Set the oven temperature at 375° F/191° C.
2. Lightly spritz a baking pan using cooking oil spray.
3. Beat the butter with both types of sugar until creamy.
4. Add the vanilla and water. Mix in the eggs individually, thoroughly mixing after adding each one.
5. Whisk the flour with the baking powder, milk powder, baking soda, salt, and cocoa. Mix it in with the creamed mixture - stirring until just combined. Lastly, mix in the bananas.
6. Scoop the mixture into the pan.
7. Bake until the cake begins to pull from the pan's sides (23-28 min.).
8. Leave it in the pan and set it aside to cool thoroughly before dusting it using a bit of confectioner' sugar to serve.

Servings Provided: 18

Time Required: 50 minutes

Macro Counts - Each Serving:

- ☐ Calories: 172
- ☐ Carbs: 29 g
- ☐ Sugar: 17 g
- ☐ Fiber: 1 g
- ☐ Chol: 33 mg
- ☐ Protein: 3 g
- ☐ Sodium: 223 mg
- ☐ Fat Content: 5 g (Saturated: 3 g)
  D.E:
- ☐ Starch: 2
- ☐ Fat: 1

Ingredients Needed:

- ☐ Unchilled butter (.33 cup)
- ☐ Eggs (2)
- ☐ Buttermilk (.5 cup)
- ☐ Sugar (1.25 cups)
- ☐ Applesauce - unsweetened (.33 cup)
- ☐ Vanilla extract (1 tsp.)
- ☐ Semisweet chocolate - melted (2 oz.)
- ☐ Bak. soda (.25 tsp.)
- ☐ A.P. flour (2.25 cups)
- ☐ Salt (1 tsp.)
- ☐ Bak. powder (1.5 tsp.)
- ☐ Shredded zucchini (2 cups)
- ☐ Confectioners' sugar (2 tsp.)
- ☐ Also Needed: 13x9-inch baking dish

Preparation Technique:

1. Use a big mixing container to cream the sugar and butter together until it crumbles (two min.).
2. Whisk and mix in the eggs. Beat in the applesauce, chocolate, buttermilk, and vanilla. Sift the baking powder with the baking soda, flour, and salt, mixing it into butter mixture just until moistened. Add in the zucchini.
3. Scoop the mixture into the baking dish coated with a spritz of baking oil spray.
4. Bake the cake at 350° Fahrenheit or 177 ° Celsius for ½ hour to 35 minutes.
5. Place it on a rack to cool and add a dusting of confectioners' sugar to serve.

Servings Provided: 12

Time Required: 1 hour 50 minutes

Macro Counts - Each Serving:

- ☐ Calories: 137
- ☐ Carbs: 26.5 g
- ☐ Sugar: 17.4 g
- ☐ Fiber: 0.2 g
- ☐ Chol: -0- mg
- ☐ Prot: 4 g
- ☐ Sodium: 42.6 mg
- ☐ Fat Content: 17.4 g (Saturated: 1.4 g)
  D.E.:
- ☐ Other Carbs: 1 ½

Ingredients Needed:

- ☐ Egg whites (1.25 cups/8-10 large eggs)
- ☐ Granulated sugar (.66 or 2/3 cup)
- ☐ A.P. flour (.75 cup)
- ☐ Cocoa powder - unsweetened (.25 cup)
- ☐ Cream of tartar (1.25 tsp.)
- ☐ Powdered sugar (.5 cup)
- ☐ Crushed instant coffee crystals/Instant espresso coffee powder (1 tbsp.)
- ☐ Vanilla extract (.5 tsp.)
- ☐ Chai-Spiced Cream (1 recipe - below)
- ☐ The Cream:
- ☐ Light whipped dessert topping - frozen (½ - 8 oz. container)
- ☐ Ground cardamom (.125 tsp.)
- ☐ Cinnamon (.125 tsp.)
- ☐ Spices @ 1 pinch each:
- ☐ Ground cloves
- ☐ Nutmeg

- ☐ Ground black pepper
- ☐ Ground ginger
- ☐ Optional: Chocolate-covered coffee beans (12)
- ☐ Also Needed: 10-inch tube pan

Preparation Technique:

1. Thaw the dessert topping.
2. Place the oven rack in the bottom position. Warm the oven temperature to 350° Fahrenheit or 177° Celsius.
3. Break and place the egg whites in a holding container on the countertop for ½ hour.
4. Sift the flour, cocoa powder, powdered sugar, and espresso powder thoroughly (3 times). You need to be sure it is lump-free.
5. Adjust the baking rack to the lowest position in the oven.
6. Use an electric mixer to blend the vanilla and cream of tartar with the egg whites using the medium-speed setting until soft peaks form.
7. Slowly add the granulated sugar (2 tbsp. at a time), once again, blending until stiff peaks are formed.
8. Sift ¼ of the flour mixture over beaten egg whites, folding it in gently. Continue folding in the rest of the flour mixture using 1/3 portions. Spoon the mixture into an ungreased pan.
9. Bake the cake until the top springs back when lightly touched (30-35 min.).
10. Promptly invert the cake into the pan and wait for it to thoroughly cool. Loosen the sides of the cake from the pan and remove it
11. Prepare the cream. Put thawed light whipped dessert topping in a medium mixing container. Add the cardamom with the black pepper, ground cloves, cinnamon, nutmeg, and ginger. Toss gently to combine.
12. Scoop the cream into 12 small portions around the edge and top of the cake. Decorate each one with a coffee bean.

Servings Provided: 16

Time Required: 55 minutes + cool time

Macro Counts - Each Serving:

- Calories: 130
- Carbs: 28 g
- Sugar: 22 g
- Prot.: 4 g
- Fat Content: -0- g
- Sodium: 116 mg
  D.E:
- Starch: 2

Ingredients Needed:

- Unchilled egg whites (12 large)
- Salt (.5 tsp.)
- Cream of tartar (1.5 tsp.)
- A.P. flour (1 cup)
- Sugar - divided (1.75 cups)
- Orange - Almond & vanilla extract (1 tsp. each)
- Orange zest (1 tsp.)
- Optional: Yellow & red food coloring (6 drops of each)
- Needed: Tube pan (10-inch)

Preparation Technique:

1. Separate the egg whites in a large mixing container for ½ hour to unchill. Grease the pan and place it to the side for now.
2. Sift or whisk the flour with the sugar (¾ cup). Set the container to the side.
3. Whisk the salt and cream of tartar with the vanilla and almond extracts - mixing them into the egg whites.

4. Use a mixer (medium-speed setting) to create soft peaks. Slowly mix in the rest of the sugar (2 tbsp. at a time), beating on high until stiff glossy peaks form and the sugar is liquified. Slowly mix in the flour mixture (½ cup portions).

5. Scoop ½ of the batter into the greased pan.

6. Mix in the orange zest with the food coloring, orange extract, and the rest of the batter. Scoop small portions of the orange batter over white batter. Swirl it using a toothpick.

7. Position the oven rack on it's lowest level. Bake at 375° Fahrenheit or 191° Celsius until browned (30-35 min.). Promptly invert the pan and thoroughly cool (1 hr.).

8. You may need to run a butter knife around the pan's edges and place the cake onto a serving plate.

Servings Provided: 24

Time Required: 35 minutes

Macro Counts - Each Serving:

- ☐ Calories: 220
- ☐ Carbs: 31g
- ☐ Fiber: 1 g
- ☐ Sugar: 22 g
- ☐ Chol: 30 mg
- ☐ Prot.: 4 g
- ☐ Sodium: 166 mg
- ☐ Fat Content: 9 g (Saturated: 4 g)
  D.E.:
- ☐ Starch: 2
- ☐ Fat: 1 ½

Ingredients Needed:

- ☐ Creamy-style peanut butter (.5 cup)
- ☐ Butter - cubed (6 tbsp.)
- ☐ Water (1 cup)
- ☐ A.P. flour (2 cups)
- ☐ Sugar (1.5 cups)
- ☐ Buttermilk (.5 cup)
- ☐ Unsweetened applesauce (.25 cup)
- ☐ Large eggs (2 lightly beaten)
- ☐ Bak. powder (1.25 tsp.)
- ☐ Vanilla extract (1 tsp.)
- ☐ Salt (.5 tsp.)
- ☐ Bak. soda (.25 tsp.)
- ☐ The Frosting:
- ☐ Butter - cubed (.25 cup)
- ☐ Peanut butter - creamy (.25 cup)

- ☐ Vanilla extract (1 tsp.)
- ☐ Milk - fat-free (2 tbsp.)
- ☐ Confectioners' sugar (1.75 cups)
- ☐ Suggested: 15x10x1-inch baking pan

Preparation Technique:

1. Prepare a large saucepan and add the peanut butter, water, and butter - just to a boil. Immediately take the pan from the burner.
2. Mix in the buttermilk, flour, eggs, applesauce, baking powder, sugar, salt, baking soda, and vanilla. Thoroughly stir until it's creamy smooth.
3. Empty the batter into the baking pan coated with a bit of cooking oil spray.
4. Set a timer and bake at 375° Fahrenheit or 191° Celsius until they are a nice brown to your liking (15-20 min.). Wait for it to cool on the countertop for 20 minutes.
5. Melt the butter and peanut butter in a saucepan using the medium temperature setting. Stir in the milk and wait for it to boil. Immediately transfer the pan from the burner.
6. Mix in the confectioners' sugar and vanilla until it's creamy smooth.
7. Spread the mixture over the warm cake. Thoroughly cool it using a wire rack.
8. Refrigerate any leftovers for another time.

Servings Provided: 16

Time Required: 55 minutes + cooling time

Macro Counts - Each Serving:

- ☐ Calories: 149
- ☐ Carbs: 28 g
- ☐ Sugar: 16 g
- ☐ Fiber: 0 g
- ☐ Chol: 12 mg
- ☐ Prot.: 2 g
- ☐ Sodium: 232 mg
- ☐ Fat Content: 3 g (Saturated: 1 g)
  D.E.:
- ☐ Starch: 2
- ☐ Fat: ½

Ingredients Needed:

- ☐ Sliced pears - reduced-sugar (15 oz. can)
- ☐ White cake mix (16.25 oz./regular size pkg.)
- ☐ Egg whites - unchilled (2 large)
- ☐ Egg- unchilled (1 large)
- ☐ Confectioners' sugar (2 tsp.)
- ☐ Pan Needed: Ten-inch fluted tube pan

Preparation Technique:

1. Drain the pears, saving the syrup.
2. Chop the pears and place them with the syrup in a big mixing container.
3. Whisk and mix the egg whites and egg with the cake mix and blend them using the low-speed setting of an electric mixer (30 sec.). Beat using the high setting for four minutes.
4. Spritz the pan with cooking oil spray and a sprinkle of flour. Add batter.
5. Bake at 350° Fahrenheit or 177 ° Celsius for 48-55 minutes.

6. Cool the cake for ten minutes before removing from the pan to a wire rack to thoroughly cool.

7. Sprinkle the cake using the sugar to serve.

Layered Cakes

Servings Provided: 1.5 dozen

Time Required: 45 minutes

Macro Counts - Each Serving:

- ☐ Calories: 83
- ☐ Carbs: 10 g
- ☐ Sugar: 5 g
- ☐ Fiber: 1 g
- ☐ Chol: 2 mg
- ☐ Prot: 2 g
- ☐ Sodium: 50 mg
- ☐ Fat Content: 4 g (Saturated: 1 g)
  D.E:
- ☐ Starch: ½
- ☐ Fat: 1
- ☐ Fruit:

Ingredients Needed:

- ☐ Shelled pistachios, toasted (.5 cup)
- ☐ Unblanched whole almonds, toasted (.25 cup)
- ☐ Sugar (1 tbsp.)
- ☐ Unchilled butter - softened (1 tbsp.)
- ☐ Ground cinnamon (.5 tsp.)
- ☐ Phyllo dough (12 sheets @ 14x9-inch each)
- ☐ Butter-flavored cooking spray
- ☐ Honey - divided (.25 cup)

Preparation Technique:

1. Warm the oven at 325° F/163° C.

2. Toss the pistachios and almonds into a food processor. Close the top and pulse the nuts until they're finely chopped. Measure and pour in the cinnamon, sugar, and butter. Securely close the lid and pulse until chopped and blended.

3. Arrange one sheet of phyllo dough on a work surface. Spray with a portion of cooking spray.

4. Continue with the second layer. Spread the nut mixture (1/3 cup) over phyllo to within one inch of sides and drizzle with one tablespoon honey.

5. Layer with two more sheets of phyllo. Be sure to spray each layer with cooking spray.

6. Roll it up, starting from the short side. Continue using the rest of the phyllo, nut mixture, and honey.

7. Slice each roll into six pieces. Place them with the seam side down onto a greased baking sheet. Lightly spritz using a baking oil spray. Bake until it's golden (16-20 min.). Drizzle with the rest of the honey to serve.

Servings Provided: 16

Time Required: 50 minutes + cool time

Macro Counts - Each Serving:

- Calories: 216
- Carbs: 28 g
- Sugar: 21 g
- Fiber: -0- g
- Chol: 40 mg
- Prot: 5 g
- Sodium: 164 mg
- Fat Content: 9 g (Saturated: 6 g)
  D.E:
- Starch: 2
- Fat: 2

Ingredients Needed:

- A.P. flour (1 cup)
- Confectioners' sugar (.75 cup)
- Baking cocoa (.25 cup)
- Salt (.125 tsp.)
- Baking soda (.125 tsp.)
- Cold butter - cubed (.5 cup)
- The Filling:
- Reduced-fat cream cheese (8 oz. pkg.)
- Condensed milk - sweetened - fat-free (14 oz. can)
- Egg - lightly beaten (1 large)
- Vanilla extract (2 tsp.)
- Needed: 8-inch square baking pan

Preparation Technique:

1. Program the oven setting 350° Fahrenheit/177 ° Celsius.

2. Sift or whisk the first five fixings. Cut in the butter until fine crumbs form (mixture will be powdery).

3. Reserve ½ cup of the mixture for the topping. Lightly press the rest of the mixture into the baking pan coated with a spritz of cooking oil spray. Bake just until set (8-10 minutes).

4. Mix the cream cheese until it's creamy. Slowly mix in the egg, vanilla, and milk, beating - just until incorporated. Dump it over the crust.

5. Set a timer and bake it for 15 minutes.

6. Sprinkle the reserved topping overfilling. Bake until filling is set (5-10 min.). Thoroughly cool on a rack. Store in the fridge.

Servings Provided: 12

Time Required: 55 minutes + chill time

Macro Counts - Each Serving:

- ☐ Calories: 169
- ☐ Carbs: 17 g
- ☐ Sugar: 14 g
- ☐ Fiber: -0- g
- ☐ Chol: 94 mg
- ☐ Prot.: 7 g
- ☐ Sodium: 95 mg
- ☐ Fat Content: 9 g (Saturated: 5 g)
  D.E:
- ☐ Fat: 2
- ☐ Starch: 1

Ingredients Needed:

- ☐ Eggs @ room temperature (4 large - separated)
- ☐ Vanilla extract (1 tsp.)
- ☐ Baking cocoa (.25 cup)
- ☐ A.P. flour (2 tbsp.)
- ☐ Salt (.125 tsp.)
- ☐ Cream of tartar (.5 tsp.)
- ☐ Confectioners' sugar - sifted - divided (.66 cup)
- ☐ The Filling:
- ☐ Mascarpone cheese (3 tbsp.)
- ☐ Ricotta cheese (15 oz. container)
- ☐ Sugar (.33 cup)
- ☐ Grated orange zest (1 tbsp.)
- ☐ Kahlua - coffee liqueur (1 tbsp.)
- ☐ Vanilla extract (.5 tsp.)
- ☐ Additional confectioners' sugar

☐ Also Needed: 15x10x1-inch baking pan

Preparation Technique:

1. Separate and add the egg whites into a bowl. Set the oven temperature at 325° F/163° C.
2. Cover the base of a greased baking pan with a parchment paper layer, and lightly grease/oil the paper.
3. Sift the flour with the cocoa and salt - twice.
4. Whisk the egg yolks in another container until slightly thickened.
5. Slowly mix in 1/3 cup confectioners' sugar (high speed) until thickened. Beat in vanilla. Fold in the cocoa mixture.
6. Mix the cream of tartar to the egg whites. Mix using the medium setting to create soft peaks. Slowly mix in the rest of the confectioners' sugar (1 tbsp. at a time). After soft glossy peaks form, fold ¼ of the whites into the batter, and the remaining whites. Pour it into the pan.
7. Bake until the top springs back when lightly touched (9-11 min.). Cover the cake using a layer of waxed paper and cool thoroughly on a wire rack.
8. Discard the waxed paper and invert the cake onto an 18-inch-long sheet of waxed paper dusted with confectioners' sugar. Peel off the layer of parchment paper.
9. In another container, mix the cheeses and sugar until blended. Stir in the Kahlua, zested orange bits, and vanilla. Spread the mixture over the cake to within ½ inch of the edges.
10. Roll it up, beginning with a short side. Trim the ends and place them on a platter with the seam side down.
11. Pop the roll into the fridge, covered, at least one hour before serving.
12. To serve, dust with confectioners' sugar.

Servings Provided: 16

Time Required: 1.25 hours + cooling time

Macro Counts - Each Serving:

- ¾ cup servings:
- Carbohydrates: 33 g
- Calories: 220
- Sugar: 18 g
- Fiber: 1 g
- Chol: 13 mg
- Prot.: 4 g
- Sodium: 325 mg
- Fat Content: 6 g (Saturated: 3 g)
  D.E:
- Starch: 2
- Fat: 1

Ingredients Needed:

- Gingerbread cake/cookie mix (14.5 oz. pkg.)
- Cold milk - fat-free (4 cups)
- Instant butterscotch pudding mix - sugar-free (4 pkg. @1 oz. each)
- Ground cinnamon (1 tsp.)
- Pumpkin (15 oz. can)
- Ground ginger - nutmeg & allspice (.25 tsp. each)
- Frozen & thawed reduced-fat whipped topping (12 oz. carton)

Preparation Technique:

1. Prepare and bake the gingerbread per the package instructions. Cool it thoroughly.
2. Crumble the cake, reserving ¼ of a cup of crumbs.
3. Whisk the milk with the pudding mixes and spices until thickened (2 min.). Stir in the pumpkin.

4. Use a glass bowl or 3.5-quart trifle to layer ¼ of the cake crumbs, ½ of the pumpkin mixture, ¼ of the cake crumbs, and ½ of the whipped topping. Make another layer.
5. Top with the last of the crumbs (step 2) and pop it into the fridge until it's time to serve.

Servings Provided: 9

Time Required: 25 minutes + chill time

Macro Counts - Each Serving:

- ☐ Calories: 177
- ☐ Carbs: 25 g
- ☐ Sugar: 18 g
- ☐ Fiber: -0- g
- ☐ Sodium: 80 mg
- ☐ Fat Content: 6 g (Saturated: 4g)
- ☐ Protein: 6 g
  D.E:
- ☐ Fat: 1
- ☐ Starch: 1
- ☐ Fat-free milk: ½

Ingredients Needed:

- ☐ Ladyfinger Cookies (24)
- ☐ Heavy whipping cream (.5 cup)
- ☐ Vanilla yogurt (2 cups)
- ☐ Milk - fat-free (1 cup)
- ☐ Strong coffee/Brewed espresso - cooled (.5 cup)
- ☐ Optional:
- ☐ Fresh raspberries
- ☐ Baking cocoa
- ☐ Suggested: 8-inch square dish

Preparation Technique:

1. Beat the cream to form stiff peaks. Fold in the yogurt. Spread about ½ cup of the cream mixture into the baking dish.
2. Use a shallow dish to combine the espresso with the milk. Quickly dip half (12) of the ladyfingers into the espresso mixture. Let the excess drip off.

3. Place them in a dish in a single layer. (You can break them to pieces as needed to fit the pan.). Add half of the remaining cream mixture and dust with cocoa.
4. Repeat the layers.
5. Pop them into the fridge, covered, for at least two hours before serving with the raspberries.

Chapter 6

Cupcake Favorites

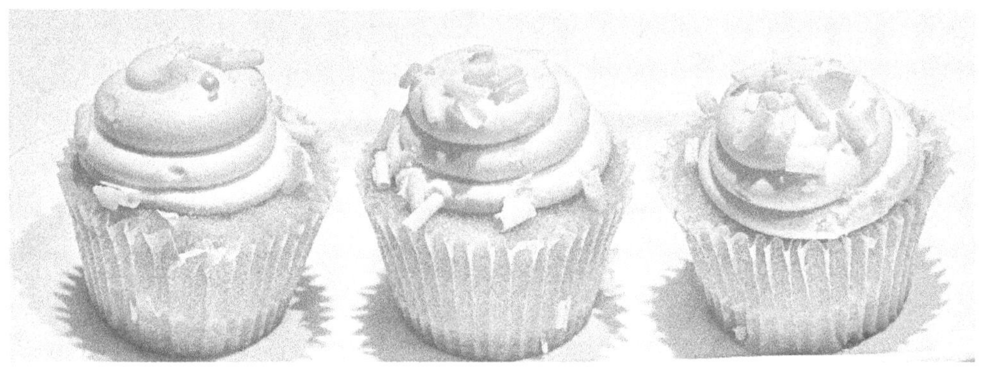

Servings Provided: 17

Time Required: 35 minutes + cool time

Macro Counts - Each Serving:

- ☐ Calories: 192
- ☐ Carbs: 33 g
- ☐ Sugar: 19 g
- ☐ Fiber: 1 g
- ☐ Chol: 22 mg
- ☐ Prot.: 3 g
- ☐ Sodium: 154 mg
- ☐ Fat Content: 5 g (Saturated: 1 g)
  D.E:
- ☐ Starch: 2
- ☐ Fat: 1

Ingredients Needed:

- ☐ Sugar (1.5 cups)
- ☐ A.P. flour (2 cups)
- ☐ Baking cocoa (.5 cup)
- ☐ Salt (.5 tsp.)
- ☐ Baking soda (1 tsp.)
- ☐ Prune baby food (.5 cup)
- ☐ Instant coffee granules (.25 cup)
- ☐ Hot water (.5 cup)
- ☐ Eggs (2)
- ☐ Canola oil (.25 cup)
- ☐ Vanilla extract (2 tsp.)
- ☐ Whipped topping - reduced-fat (1.5 cups)
- ☐ Additional baking cocoa

Preparation Technique:

1. Place paper liners in the muffin cups.
2. Sift or whisk the flour with baking soda, sugar, cocoa, and salt.
3. Dissolve the coffee in hot water. Set aside.
4. Whisk the eggs with the oil, vanilla, baby food, and coffee mixture. Gradually stir into the dry fixings - just until moistened. Fill the cups 2/3 full.
5. Bake at 350° Fahrenheit or 177 ° Celsius until a toothpick comes out clean (18-20 min.).
6. Cool them for ten minutes. Then remove them from the pans to the countertop on racks to thoroughly cool.
7. Ice the cupcakes with whipped topping and a sprinkle of cocoa right before serving. Refrigerate the leftovers for later.

Servings Provided: 1.5 dozen

Time Required: 50 minutes + cooling time

Macro Counts - Each Serving:

- ☐ Calories: 110
- ☐ Carbs: 22 g
- ☐ Sugar: 17 g
- ☐ Fiber: 1 g
- ☐ Chol: -0- mg
- ☐ Prot.: 2 g
- ☐ Sodium: 78 mg
- ☐ Fat Content: 2 g (Saturated: 2 g)
  D.E:
- ☐ Starch: 1 ½

Ingredients Needed:

- ☐ Unchilled egg whites (6 large)
- ☐ A.P. flour (.66 or 2/3 cup)
- ☐ Baking cocoa (.25 cup)
- ☐ Sugar - divided (1.33 cups)
- ☐ Baking powder (.5 tsp.)
- ☐ Almond extract (1 tsp.)
- ☐ Cream of tartar (.5 tsp.)
- ☐ Sweetened shredded coconut (1 cup)
- ☐ Salt (.25 tsp.)
- ☐ Confectioners' sugar - optional
- ☐ Muffin tin and 18 cupcake liners

Preparation Technique:

1. Break and add the egg whites into a large mixing container.
2. Set the oven temperature at 350° F/177 ° C.
3. Whisk or sift the flour with the baking powder, cocoa, and one cup of sugar twice.

4. Mix in the cream of tartar, almond extract, and salt to the egg whites. Use the mixer (medium-speed setting) to create soft peaks.

5. Slowly mix in the rest of the sugar (one tablespoon at a time) using high speed to combine them (beating after adding each one) until sugar is liquified.

6. Continue beating to form stiff glossy peaks. Slowly fold in the flour mixture (½ cup at a time). Gently fold in coconut.

7. Fill the cups 2/3 full. Bake until the top appears dry (30-35 min.).

8. Cool them in the pans for about ten minutes before transferring the cupcakes onto wire racks to cool the rest of the way. Sprinkle them using a bit of confectioner' sugar as desired.

Servings Provided: 1.5 dozen

Time Required: 50 minutes + cool time

Macro Counts - Each Serving:

- Calories: 126
- Carbs: 24 g
- Sugar: 16 g
- Fiber: 1 g
- Chol: 14 mg
- Prot.: 4 g
- Sodium: 85 mg
- Fat Content: 2 g (Saturated: 1 g)
  D.E:
- Starch: 1 ½

Ingredients Needed:

- Egg whites (2 large)
- Unchilled egg (1 large)
- Vanilla extract (1 tsp.)
- Unsweetened applesauce (.33 cup)
  ****
- A.P. flour (1.25 cups)
- Baking cocoa (.33 cup)
- Sugar (1 cup)
- Baking soda (.5 tsp.)
- Buttermilk (.75 cup)
- The Filling:
- Ricotta cheese - reduced-fat (1 cup)
- Sugar (.25 cup)
- Egg white (1 large)
- Sweetened shredded coconut (.33 cup)
- Coconut or almond extract (.5 tsp.)

☐ Confectioners' sugar

Preparation Technique:

1. Warm the oven to reach 350° Fahrenheit/177 ° Celsius.
2. Coat 18 muffin cups with cooking spray.
3. Beat the first four ingredients (up to the line **) until well blended.
4. In another mixing container, whisk the flour, cocoa, baking soda, and sugar. Slowly beat into egg mixture alternately with the buttermilk.
5. Prepare the filling by beating the ricotta cheese with the egg white and sugar until it's incorporated. Mix in the coconut and extract.
6. Fill prepared cups with half of the batter. Drop the filling by tablespoonfuls into the center of each cupcake and cover with the remainder of the batter.
7. Bake them until nicely browned (27-33 min.).
8. Let them cool for ten minutes before transferring them to wire racks to finish cooling.
9. Serve with a dusting of confectioners' sugar.

Servings Provided: 2 dozen

Time Required: 55 minutes + cool time

Macro Counts - Each Serving:

- ☐ Calories: 153
- ☐ Carbs: 25g
- ☐ Sugar: 16g
- ☐ Fiber: -0- g
- ☐ Sodium: 176 mg
- ☐ Chol: 28 mg
- ☐ Fat Content: 5 g (Saturated: 1 g)
- ☐ Protein: 2 g
  D.E:
- ☐ Starch: 1 ½
- ☐ Fat: 1 ½

Ingredients Needed:

- ☐ Lemon cake mix (regular size pkg.)
- ☐ Water (1-1/3 cups)
- ☐ Lemon creme pie filling (1 cup)
- ☐ Canola oil (1/3 cup)
- ☐ Unchilled eggs (3 large)
- ☐ Grated lemon zest (1 tbsp.)
- ☐ The Meringue:
- ☐ Unchilled egg whites (3 large)
- ☐ Sugar (.5 cup)
- ☐ Cream of tartar (.5 tsp.)

Preparation Technique:

1. Mix the cake mix with the oil, water, lemon zest, and eggs. Beat on low speed for ½ minute. Adjust the setting to medium for two minutes.
2. Fill 24 paper-lined muffin cups until they are approximately 2/3 of the way to full.

3. Bake at 350° Fahrenheit/177 ° Celsius until they are a nice brown (18-22 min.).

4. Snip a small hole in the corner of a plastic bag or use a pastry injector and insert a tiny tip. Fill it with the pie filling. Push the tip/end into the top of each cupcake to fill.

5. Whisk the egg whites with the cream of tartar using the medium-speed setting to create soft peaks.

6. Slowly mix in the sugar (1 tbsp. @ a time). Mix using the high-speed setting until stiff glossy peaks are formed, and the sugar is liquified. Pipe it over the tops of cupcakes.

7. Bake at 400° Fahrenheit/204° Celsius until the meringue is lightly browned (5-8 min.).

8. Cool the cupcakes for ten minutes in the pans. Then, move them to wire racks to cool thoroughly.

9. Keep the container in the fridge to enjoy as desired.

Chapter 7

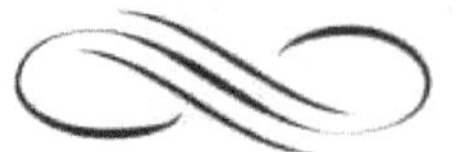

Pie & Cheesecake Favorites

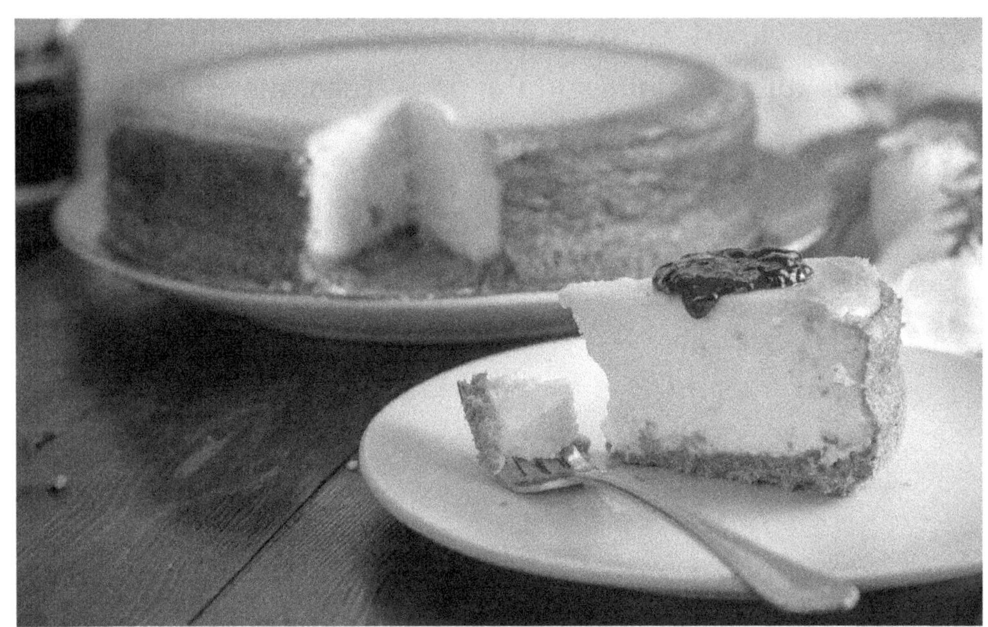

Pie Choices

Servings Provided: 4

Time Required: 20 minutes

Macro Counts - Each Serving:

- Calories: 153
- Carbs: 20 g
- Sugar: 10 g
- Fiber: 6 g
- Chol: 18 mg
- Prot.: 2 g
- Sodium: 109 mg

- Fat Content: 8 g (Saturated: 4 g)

  D.E.:
- Starch: ½
- Fat: 1 ½
- Fruit: 1

Ingredients Needed:

- Fresh raspberries (2-2/3 cups)
- Melted butter (2 tbsp.)
- Sugar (2 tsp.)
- Graham cracker crumbs (.5 cup)
- Whipped cream in a can (4 tbsp.)
- Baking cocoa (.25 tsp.)
- Also Needed: 8x6-in. rectangle baking dish

Preparation Technique:

- Toss the sugar with the raspberries and set aside for now.
- Use a separate mixing container to combine the butter with the cracker crumbs. Press the mixture into the ungreased baking sheet.
- Bake at 350° Fahrenheit/177 ° Celsius until they are browned to your liking (5-6 min.). Cool them thoroughly on a wire rack before breaking them into large chunks.
- Portion ½ of the graham cracker pieces into four dessert dishes; top with raspberries (1/3 cup).
- Continue the layers, topping each one with one tablespoon of whipped cream and a sprinkle of cocoa.

Servings Provided: 8

Time Required: 20 minutes + chill time

Macro Counts - Each Serving:

- ☐ Calories: 194
- ☐ Carbs: 33 g
- ☐ Sugar: 18 g
- ☐ Chol: 2 mg
- ☐ Prot.: 3 g
- ☐ Sodium: 159 mg
- ☐ Fat Content: 3 g (Saturated: 1 g)
  D.E:
- ☐ Starch: 2
- ☐ Fat: ½

Ingredients Needed:

- ☐ Boiling water (.25 cup)
- ☐ Sugar-free lime gelatin (0.3 oz. pkg.)
- ☐ Key lime yogurt (2 cartons @ 6 oz. each)
- ☐ Frozen & thawed fat-free whipped topping (8 oz. carton)
- ☐ Graham cracker crust - reduced-fat (8-inch)

Preparation Technique:

1. Prepare a big mixing container and add boiling water to the gelatin. Whisk it for two minutes until it is liquified.
2. Whisk in the yogurt and gently fold in the whipped topping. Dump it into the crust.
3. Pop it into the fridge with a cover until it's set (2 hrs.).

Servings Provided: 8

Time Required: 20 minutes + chill time

Macro Counts - Each Serving:

- Calories: 202
- Carbs: 30 g
- Sugar: 17 g
- Fiber: 2 g
- Chol: -0- mg
- Protein: 3 g
- Fat Content: 8 g (Saturated: 1 g)
- Sodium: 152 mg
  D.E:
- Starch: 1
- Fat: 1 ½
- Fruit: 1

Ingredients Needed:

- Ground cinnamon (.5 tsp.)
- S.F. lemon gelatin (0.3 oz. pkg.)
- Ground nutmeg (.25 tsp.)
- Water - divided (.1.75 cups)
- Tart apples (5 medium - peeled and sliced)
- S. F. - cook-&-serve vanilla pudding mix (0.8 oz. pkg.)
- Chopped nuts (.5 cup)
- Graham cracker crust - reduced-fat (6 oz.)
- Optional: Whipped topping

Preparation Technique:

1. Combine the gelatin with the nutmeg, cinnamon, and 1.5 cups water. Add the apples into a large saucepan. Wait for it to boil. Adjust the temperature setting to simmer, covered, until apples are tender (5 min.).

2. Whisk the pudding mix and the rest of the water. Stir it into the apple mixture. Cook until thickened, occasionally stirring (1 min.).
3. Remove the pan and mix in the nuts. Add it to the prepared crust.
4. Refrigerate at least two hours before serving with whipped topping or as desired.

Servings Provided: 8

Time Required: 20 minutes + chill time

Macro Counts - Each Serving:

- Calories: 184
- Carbs: 32 g
- Fiber: 1 g
- Sugar: 13 g
- Chol: 2 mg
- Protein: 6 g
- Sodium: 427 mg
- Fat Content: 3 g (Saturated: 1 g)
  D.E:
- Starch: 2
- Fat: 1

Ingredients Needed:

- Cold fat-free milk - divided (4 cups)
- Sugar-free instant vanilla pudding mix (1 oz. pkg.)
- Reduced-fat graham cracker crust (6 oz.)
- S.F. instant butterscotch pudding mix (1 oz. pkg.)
- S.F. instant chocolate pudding mix (1.4 oz. pkg.)
  Optional:
- Whipped topping
- Finely chopped pecans

Preparation Technique:

1. Whisk the milk (1.33 cups) and vanilla pudding mix for two minutes. Spread into crust.
2. In a separate mixing container, whisk another 1.33 cups of milk with the butterscotch pudding mix for two minutes. Carefully spoon over the vanilla layer, spreading evenly.
3. Use another container to whisk the rest of the milk (1.33 cups) and chocolate pudding. Mix for two minutes. Carefully spread over the top.

4. Refrigerate until set, at least ½ hour.

5. Top it off using whipped topping and pecans to your liking.

Servings Provided: 8

Time Required: 15 minutes + chill time

Macro Counts - Each Serving:

- Calories: 185
- Carbs: 27 g
- Sugar: 14 g
- Prot.: 1 g
- Sodium: 275 mg
- Fat Content: 8 g (Saturated: 4 g)
  D.E:
- Starch: 2
- Fat: 1

Ingredients Needed:

- Reduced-fat whipped topping -frozen & thawed - divided (8 oz. carton)
- Diet root beer - cold (.75 cup)
- Fat-free milk (.5 cup)
- Instant vanilla pudding mix - sugar-free (1 oz. pkg.)
- Graham cracker crust (9-inch crust/about 6 oz.)
- Optional: Maraschino cherries

Preparation Technique:

1. Set aside and refrigerate ½ cup whipped topping for garnish.
2. Whisk the milk with the root beer and pudding to mix for two minutes.
3. Mix in ½ of the remaining whipped topping.
4. Spread the remainder of whipped topping over the pie. Freeze overnight or at least eight hours.
5. Scoop the reserved whipped topping over each serving and garnish using a maraschino cherry if desired.
6. Note: It's also delicious from the freezer!

Servings Provided: 8

Time Required: 40 minutes

Macro Counts - Each Serving:

- ☐ Calories: 174
- ☐ Carbs: 25 g
- ☐ Sugar: 16 g
- ☐ Fiber: 2 g
- ☐ Chol: 26 mg
- ☐ Protein: 5 g
- ☐ Sodium: 207 mg
- ☐ Fat Content: 7 g (Saturated: 1 g)
  D.E:
- ☐ Starch: 1 ½
- ☐ Fat: 1

Ingredients Needed:

- ☐ Tart apples - chopped (2 medium)
- ☐ Whole wheat flour (.25 cup)
- ☐ Salt (.5 tsp.)
- ☐ Baking powder (1 tsp.)
- ☐ A.P. flour (.25 cup)
- ☐ Sugar (.5 cup)
- ☐ Ground cinnamon (.5 tsp.)
- ☐ Egg (1 large)
- ☐ Vanilla extract (.25 tsp.)
- ☐ Chopped - toasted pecans or walnuts (.75 cup)
- ☐ Optional: Confectioners' sugar
- ☐ Also Needed: 9-inch pie plate

Preparation Technique:

1. Warm the oven at 350° Fahrenheit or 177 ° Celsius.

2. Sift each type of flour with salt, sugar, cinnamon, and baking powder.
3. Beat the egg with the vanilla. Mix them into the dry components - just until moistened. Fold in walnuts and apples.
4. Pour it into the pie plate coated with a spritz of baking oil spray.
5. Bake them for 25-30 minutes.
6. Dust it using confectioners' sugar as desired and serve warm.

Cheesecake Choices

Servings Provided: 12

Time Required: 4 hours 55 minutes

Macro Counts - Each Serving:

- Calories: 176
- Carbs: 14 g
- Sugar: 7 g
- Fiber: 1 g
- Chol: 28 mg
- Protein: 6 g
- Sodium: 236 mg
- Fat Content: 11 g (Saturated: 7 g)
  D.E.:
- Fat: 2
- Other Carbohydrate: 1

Ingredients Needed:

- Small pretzel twists (1.5 cups/2 oz.)
- Sliced almonds - toasted (2 tbsp.)
- Melted butter (3 tbsp.)
- Water (.33 cup)
- Unflavored gelatin (1 envelope)
- Unchilled reduced-fat cream cheese (12 oz.)
- R.F. sour cream (8 oz.)
- Confectioners' sugar (.25 cup)
- Almond extract (.5 tsp.)
- Frozen - Light whipped dessert topping - thawed (4 oz.)
- Fresh strawberries - divided (1 cup)
- Fresh blackberries or blueberries - divided (1 cup)

Preparation Technique:

1. Quarter and slice the berries into halves.

2. Toss the almonds and pretzels into a food processor.

3. Place the lid on it and pulse them until finely crushed.

4. Add butter and replace the top, and pulse the mixture thoroughly to combine.

5. Press the pretzel mixture into the bottom of an eight or nine-inch springform pan.

6. Bake until lightly browned (8 to 10 min.). Cool on a wire rack.

7. Pour the water into a saucepan. Add the gelatin (don't stir). Let it soften for about five minutes.

8. Cook and stir using the low-temperature setting until the gelatin liquefies. Let it cool slightly.

9. Use an electric mixer - using the medium setting - to combine the sour cream, cream cheese, almond extract, and confectioners' sugar. Add the gelatin mixture and beat until combined. Mix in the whipped topping.

10. Spread ½ of the filling over the cooled crust, adding ½ of the strawberries blackberries.

11. Scoop and add the remainder of the cream cheese mixture over the berries.

12. Use a layer of foil or plastic to cover the cake.

13. Chill it until set (for 4-24 hrs.).

14. Loosen the cake when removing it from the pan using a sharp knife around the edges.

15. Pop away the sides of the pan and slice the cheesecake into wedges.

16. Garnish each portion with the rest of the berries as desired.

Servings Provided: 12

Time Required: 4 hours 45 minutes

Macro Counts - Each Serving:

- ☐ Calories: 156
- ☐ Carbs: 18.9 g
- ☐ Fiber: 0.7 g
- ☐ Sugar: 15 g
- ☐ Chol: 17.3 mg
- ☐ Protein: 4.4 g
- ☐ Sodium: 147.4 mg
- ☐ Fat Content: 7.6 g (Saturated: 4.5 g)
  D.E.:
- ☐ Other Carbohydrate: 1
- ☐ Fat: 1 ½

Ingredients Needed:

- ☐ Reduced-fat vanilla wafers (12)
- ☐ R.F Unchilled cream cheese (8 oz. pkg.)
- ☐ Unchilled fat-free cream cheese (½ of an 8 oz.pkg.)
- ☐ Bittersweet/semisweet chocolate - melted & cooled (3 oz.)
- ☐ Sugar (.5 cup)
- ☐ Nonfat milk (.25 cup)
- ☐ Vanilla extract (1.5 tsp.)
- ☐ Egg white - lightly beaten (1 large)
- ☐ Dried cherries or dried apricots (.25 cup)
- ☐ Chocolate curls and/or small whole or sliced strawberries (1 oz.)
- ☐ Requested: Twelve 2.5-inch muffin cups

Preparation Technique:

1. Warm the oven to 350° Fahrenheit or 177 ° Celsius.
2. Line the cups with foil or paper bake cups. Place one wafer into each cup.

3. Beat both types of cream cheese in a mixing container using an electric mixer (medium-speed setting for ½ minute).
4. Blend in the sugar, chocolate, milk, and vanilla until thoroughly incorporated. Stir in the egg white. Finely chop and add the dried cherries/apricots. Scoop the filling into the prepared cups (3/4 full).
5. Bake until set (20 min.). Let them cool in the pan for five minutes.
6. Transfer the cheesecakes from the pan. Cool on a wire rack for about one hour.
7. Place a layer of foil or plastic wrap over the cake. Let it chill for three hours or as long as 24 hours.
8. If you like, garnish with chocolate curls or strawberries before serving.

Servings Provided: 12

Time Required: 70 minutes + chill time

Macro Counts - Each Serving:

- ☐ Calories: 187
- ☐ Carbs: 17 g
- ☐ Sugar: 14 g
- ☐ Fiber: 1 g
- ☐ Chol: 46 mg
- ☐ Prot.: 8 g
- ☐ Sodium: 378 mg
- ☐ Fat Content: 8 g (Saturated: 5 g)
  D.E:
- ☐ Starch: 1 ½
- ☐ Fat: ½
- ☐ Lean Meat: 1

Ingredients Needed:

- ☐ 2% cottage cheese (2 cups)
- ☐ Crushed chocolate wafers (1 cup/about 16 wafers)
- ☐ Reduced-fat cream cheese, cubed (8 oz. pkg.)
- ☐ Sugar (.5 cup)
- ☐ Salt (1 dash)
- ☐ Vanilla extract (1 tbsp.)
- ☐ Eggs (2 large)
- ☐ Egg white (1 large)
- ☐ Bittersweet chocolate (2 oz.)
- ☐ Optional: Fresh raspberries
- ☐ Also Needed:
- ☐ 9-inch springform pan & baking tray
- ☐ Foil (2 sheets @ 18-inches square)

Preparation Technique:

1. Line a strainer with one coffee filter or four layers of cheesecloth. Place it over a bowl. Add the cottage cheese into the strainer, refrigerate, and cover for one hour.
2. Place the springform pan over the doubled foil and wrap foil securely around the pan.
3. Spritz the inside of the pan with cooking oil spray. Press crushed wafers over the bottom and one inch up its sides.
4. Set the oven to 350° Fahrenheit or 177 ° Celsius.
5. Pulse the drained cottage cheese in a food processor until it is creamy. Measure and mix in the salt, cream cheese, and sugar, processing until blended.
6. Empty the mixture into a mixing container and whisk in the vanilla, eggs, and egg white. Add one cup of batter into a small dish and fold in the melted chocolate.
7. Empty the plain batter into the crust. Then, drop chocolate batter by spoonfuls over the plain batter. Swirl the batter with a skewer or knife. Arrange the springform pan into a larger baking pan; add one inch of boiling water to a larger pan.
8. Set a timer and bake until the center is just set (40 min.).
9. Turn off the heat in the oven and slightly open the door. Cool the cheesecake in the oven for ½ hour.
10. Transfer the springform pan from the water bath. Remove the foil. Loosen sides of cheesecake with a knife; cool on a wire rack for ½ hour. Once it's thoroughly cooled, cover and pop it into the fridge overnight.
11. Remove the rim from the pan and top with raspberries.

Servings Provided: 12

Time Required: 45 minutes + cooling times

Macro Counts - Each Serving:

- ☐ Calories: 244
- ☐ Carbs: 29 g
- ☐ Sugar: 17 g
- ☐ Fiber: 2 g
- ☐ Chol: 16 mg
- ☐ Protein: 10 g
- ☐ Sodium: 463 mg
- ☐ Fat Content: 8 g (Saturated: 5 g)
  D.E.:
- ☐ Starch: 2
- ☐ Fat: 1 ½

Ingredients Needed:

- ☐ Chocolate graham cracker crumbs (1.25 cups/8-9 crackers)
- ☐ Melted butter (.25 cup)
- ☐ Unflavored gelatin (2 envelopes)
- ☐ Cold-water (.5 cup)
- ☐ Fresh/frozen - unsweetened strawberries - thawed (16 oz.)
- ☐ F.F. cream cheese - cubed (2 pkg. @ 8 ounces of each)
- ☐ Cottage cheese - fat-free (1 cup)
- ☐ Sugar substitute (equal to .75 cup sugar)
- ☐ Reduced-fat whipped topping - frozen & thawed - divided (8 oz. carton)
- ☐ Chocolate ice cream topping (.5 cup)
- ☐ Quartered fresh strawberries (1 cup)
- ☐ Also Needed: 9-inch springform pan

Preparation Technique:

1. Warm the oven to 350° Fahrenheit or 177° Celsius.

2. Combine the butter with the cracker crumbs. Push the crust mixture into the bottom and one inch up the sides of the baking pan coated with cooking spray.

3. Put the pan on a baking tray to bake until set (ten minutes). Thoroughly cool it on a wire rack.

4. Add the gelatin into cold water in a saucepan. Wait for about one minute. Warm it using the low-temperature setting, stirring until the gelatin is completely liquified. Remove the pan from the hot burner.

5. Remove the strawberry hulls and puree the berries in a food processor. Pour it into a mixing container and combine the cottage cheese with the cream cheese and sugar substitute into the food processor, processing until smooth. While processing, gradually add in the gelatin mixture.

6. Mix in the pureed strawberries and process until thoroughly mixed.

7. Transfer the berries into a large mixing container and fold in two cups whipped topping. Scoop it into the crust.

8. Place a layer over it and pop it into the fridge until set (two to three hrs.)

9. Use a butter knife to loosen the sides of the cheesecake and remove the rim.

10. Garnish the cake using the chocolate topping, the rest of the whipped topping, and the deliciously quartered strawberries.

Servings Provided: 12

Time Required: 1 hour 50 minutes

Macro Counts - Each Serving:

- ☐ Calories: 124
- ☐ Carbs: 15.4 g
- ☐ Sugar: 10.7 g
- ☐ Fiber: 0.2 g
- ☐ Chol: 14 mg
- ☐ Sodium: 143.4 mg
- ☐ Fat Content: 5.1 g (Saturated: 2.4 g)
  D.E.:
- ☐ Starch: 1
- ☐ Fat: 1

Ingredients Needed:

- ☐ Nonstick cooking spray
- ☐ Gingersnap cookies, such as Nabisco® brand (15 @ 2-inches each)
- ☐ Reduced-fat cream cheese - ex. - Neufchâtel (8 oz. pkg.)
- ☐ Pineapple F.F. Greek yogurt (6 oz. container)
- ☐ Sugar substitute (2 tbsp.)**
- ☐ A.P. flour (1 tbsp.)
- ☐ Vanilla (1 tsp.)
- ☐ Ground ginger (.75 tsp.)
- ☐ Refrigerated or frozen egg product, thawed (6 tbsp.)
- ☐ Crushed pineapple - juice pack (8 oz. can)
- ☐ Finely chopped, crystallized ginger (2 tbsp.)
- ☐ Also Needed: 12-count muffin tin

Preparation Technique:

1. Preheat the oven to 350° Fahrenheit/177 ° Celsius. Drain the pineapple.

2. Line the cups with paper liners. Spray the paper bake cups using a spritz of cooking spray.
3. Add one gingersnap cookie into the bottom of each of the cups.
4. Finely crush the final three gingersnap cookies and set aside.
5. Blend the cream cheese with an electric mixer using the medium-speed setting until smooth.
6. Add the yogurt, sugar, flour, vanilla, and ground ginger, beating until combined.
7. Mix in the egg, drained pineapple, and one tablespoon of the crystallized ginger.
8. Portion the batter between the prepared bake cups. Sprinkle the last tablespoon of crystallized ginger and the reserved crushed gingersnaps over the batter in each of the cups.
9. Bake them for about 15 minutes until cheesecakes appear set. Cool in the muffin cups for 20 minutes.
10. Remove cheesecakes from the cups and cool thoroughly using a wire rack. Cover and chill them for one to four hours.
11. To serve, remove each of the cheesecakes from the paper bake cups to serve.
12. Note** The substitute should be equivalent to two tablespoons of sugar.

Servings Provided: 25

Time Required: 9 hours 35 minutes

Macro Counts - Each Serving:

- Calories: 142
- Carbs: 14.8g
- Fiber: 0.2 g
- Sugar: 10.4 g
- Chol: 40.7 mg
- Prot.: 4.8 g
- Sodium: 244.4 mg
- Fat Content: 7.2 g (Saturated: 3.8 g)
  D.E.:
- Fat: 1 ½
- Other Carbohydrate: ½

Ingredients Needed:

- Graham crackers (1 cup)
- Sugar (1 cup)
- Butter (3 tbsp.)
- Milk - fat-free (1 cup)
- F.F & sugar-free lemon instant pudding mix (1 cup/4-serving-size pkg.)
- Unchilled reduced-fat cream cheese - Neufchâtel (2 - 8 oz. packs)
- F.F. cream cheese - softened (8 oz. pkg.)
- Plain fat-free Greek yogurt (.25 cup)
- Salt (.25 tsp.)
- Eggs (3)
- Lemon peel (2 tbsp.)
- Lemon juice (2 tbsp.)
- White baking pieces (2 tbsp.)
- Shortening (.5 tsp.)
- Chopped pistachio nuts (2 tbsp.)

☐ Also Needed: 9x9x2-inch baking pan

Preparation Technique:

1. Set the oven temperature to 325° F/163° C.
2. Cover the baking tray using a layer of foil, making sure to also cover the pan's edges.
3. Finely crush the crackers and shred the lemon peel. Melt the butter.
4. Combine the crushed crackers, ¼ cup of the sugar, and the butter. Evenly push it into the prepared pan. Bake for ten minutes, then cool on a wire rack.
5. Whisk the milk with the pudding mix until smooth and set aside.
6. Beat Neufchatel cheese with the cream cheese using an electric mixer (medium-high speed setting) for ½ minute.
7. Mix in the rest of the sugar (¾ cup) with the yogurt, salt, and pudding mixture. Beat until combined.
8. Break in the eggs, mixing after each addition. Mix in one tablespoon of the lemon peel and the lemon juice until incorporated. Scoop the batter over the cooled crust.
9. Bake until a one-inch area around the outside edges appears set when gently shaken (1-1 ¼ hrs.).
10. Thoroughly cool it in the pan on a rack. Cover the cheesecake using a plastic wrap, making sure the plastic wrap touches the surface of the cheesecake to avoid condensation. Chill for a minimum of eight hours or up to one day.
11. Toss the white baking pieces and shortening into a microwave-safe bowl and melt (high @ 100% power) for 10 seconds to one minute. Stir it every 20 seconds.
12. Sprinkle it over the cheesecake with chopped pistachios.
13. Lift the cake from the pan and slice into squares.
14. Garnish the cheesecake using the rest of the lemon peel (1 tbsp.). Serve as desired.

Servings Provided: 12

Time Required: 3 hours 35 minutes

Macro Counts - Each Serving:

- Calories: 202
- Carbs: 18.9 g
- Fiber: 0.5 g
- Sugar: 13.3 g
- Chol: 35.6 mg
- Protein: 4.6 g
- Sodium: 206.1 mg
- Fat Content: 12.4 g (Saturated: 6.9 g)
  D.E.:
- Starch: 1
- Fat: 2 ½

Ingredients Needed:

- Cooking oil spray (as needed)
- Gingersnaps (15 crumbled)
- Melted butter (3 tbsp.)
- Sugar (2 tbsp. + .33 cup)
- Unflavored gelatin (1 envelope)
- Boiling water (1 cup)
- Unchilled R.F. cream cheese - Neufchatel (2 - 8 oz. pkg.)
- Vanilla (1 tsp.)
- Lime juice (1 tbsp.)
- Medium ripened mango (1)
- Suggested: 9-inch pie plate/8-inch springform pan

Preparation Technique:

1. Lightly coat the baking container with cooking spray; set aside.

2. Finely grind the gingersnaps in a food processor. Melt and pour in the butter with two tablespoons of sugar while the mixer is running. Process the mixture until the crumbs are moistened.

3. Empty the mixture into the prepared pan, pushing it over the bottom and one inch up the baking pan's sides.

4. Whisk the gelatin with the sugar (1/3 cup). Pour in boiling water, stirring until the gelatin is liquified (5 min.).

5. Combine the vanilla with the cream cheese using the medium-speed setting of an electric mixer. Slowly mix in the gelatin mixture. Empty the mixture into the crust.

6. Peel, remove the seeds, and chop the mango; toss it into a food processor with the lime juice. Place a lid on the blender and mix until it's a smooth puree. Push the mango puree through a fine-mesh sieve and discard solids.

7. Drizzle three tablespoons of the mango puree over the cheesecake filling. Swirl it with a knife to create a marbled effect. Place a layer of foil over the cake and pop it into the fridge to chill. Add the remaining mango puree and chill for another three hours or until the cheesecake is firm.

8. To serve, discard the pan's sides and slice cheesecake into wedges.

9. Serve the remaining mango puree with cheesecake wedges or any way you desire.

Servings Provided: 12

Time Required: 8 hours 35 minutes

Macro Counts - Each Serving:

- ☐ Calories: 148
- ☐ Carbs: 12.2 g
- ☐ Fiber: 1.3 g
- ☐ Sugar: 2.6 g
- ☐ Chol: 22.7 mg
- ☐ Protein: 8.9 g
- ☐ Sodium: 330.9 mg
- ☐ Fat Content: 7.4 g (Saturated: 4.5 g)
  D.E.:
- ☐ Fat: 1 ½
- ☐ Other Carbs: 1 ½

Ingredients Needed:

- ☐ Graham crackers (.75 cup)
- ☐ Butter (2 tbsp.)
- ☐ Cream cheese -reduced-fat - Neufchâtel (8 oz. pkg.)
- ☐ Sugar (.5 cup)
- ☐ Milk - fat-free (.5 cup)
- ☐ Grated orange peel (.5 tsp.)
- ☐ Vanilla (2 tsp.)
- ☐ F.F cream cheese (2 @ 8 oz. pkg.)
- ☐ Pumpkin (15 oz. can)
- ☐ Pumpkin pie spice (1 tsp.)
- ☐ Orange juice (.25 cup)
- ☐ Unflavored gelatin (.25 oz. envelope)
- ☐ Also Needed: 8-inch springform baking pan

Preparation Technique:

1. First, melt the butter. Finely crush and combine the crackers with the butter until the crackers are moistened. Push the crust mixture onto the bottom of the pan. Use a layer of plastic and cover the pan. Chill while you prepare the filling.

2. Use a blender/food processor to combine ¼ cup of sugar, cream cheese, ¼ cup of milk, orange peel, and vanilla. Place a lid on the blender and mix until it's creamy smooth. Transfer the mixture into a holding container and put it to the side for now.

3. Next, combine the pumpkin with the remaining ¼ cup milk, the fat-free cream cheese, the rest of the ¼ cup sugar, and the pumpkin pie spice. Securely close the lid and blend until smooth.

4. Sprinkle the gelatin into the orange juice into a pan and let it marinate for five minutes. Simmer and stir using the low-temperature setting until the gelatin is liquified.

5. Combine one tablespoon of the gelatin mixture into the white cream cheese mixture and the remainder of the gelatin mixture into the pumpkin mixture.

6. Empty the pumpkin mixture over the chilled crust. Slowly empty the white cream cheese mixture over the pumpkin mixture. Swirl the pumpkin and white blends.

7. Use a layer of foil to chill the cake overnight before serving.

8. Gently 'break' the cheesecake from the sides of the pan and pop it out. Slice it into wedges to serve.

Servings Provided: 10

Time Required: 4 hours 50 minutes

Macro Counts - Each Serving:

- Calories: 137
- Carbs: 15.8 g
- Sugar: 8.5 g
- Fiber: 1.1 g
- Chol: 14 mg
- Prot.: 4.3 g
- Sodium: 159.4 mg
- Fat Content: 6.2 g (Saturated: 4.2 g)
  D.E.:
- Fat: 1
- Other Carbohydrate: 1

Ingredients Needed:

- Frozen phyllo dough - thawed (8 sheets)
- Toasted wheat germ (3 tbsp.)
- Water (3 tbsp.)
- Unflavored gelatin (1.5 tsp.)
- Light cream cheese - softened (8 oz. pkg.)
- Light dairy sour cream (.5 cup)
- Powdered sugar (1 tbsp.)
- Frozen light whipped dessert topping (half of 8 oz. container)
- Assorted melon pieces (3 cups)
- Fresh raspberries (.25 cup)
- Fresh thyme and/or oregano (1 sprig)
- Butter-flavor nonstick cooking spray (as needed)
- Non-stick cooking oil spray (as needed)
- Suggested: 9-inch tart pan with a removable bottom (1 to 2 inches deep)

Preparation Technique:

1. Thaw the whipped topping.
2. Thinly slice the melon into wedges - removing the peel.
3. Coat the tart pan using a nonstick cooking spray.
4. Tip: While you are preparing each of the tarts, cover the rest of the sheets with a plastic wrap to keep them fresh.
5. Remove a sheet from the package of dough. Lightly spritz it with the cooking spray.
6. Add another sheet of the phyllo dough and also spray it.
7. Gently push the dough into the tart pan, extending it to the edge of the pan. Dust the crust with the wheat germ (1 tbsp.).
8. Lightly spray and layer another two sheets of the dough, placing it across the phyllo in the pan (criss-cross fashion). Sprinkle using another tablespoon of the wheat germ.
9. Add two more sheets of the phyllo dough, cooking spray, and wheat germ, placing the rectangles in the pan at an angle to completely cover the bottom of the pan.
10. Once more, add the last two sheets of dough and nonstick cooking spray. Turn under the edges of phyllo dough to form a border.Bake until the crust is lightly browned (10-12 min.). Cool in a pan on a wire rack.
11. Prepare the filling: Pour the water into the pan and add the gelatin (*don't stir*). Wait for five minutes until it softens.
12. Cook and stir using the low-temperature setting until the gelatin liquefies. Wait for it to slightly cool.
13. Use the medium-speed setting of an electric mixer to beat the sour cream with the cream cheese and powdered sugar until smooth. Add in the gelatin mixture, pulsing until combined. Lastly, mix in the whipped topping.
14. Scoop the batter into the cooled crust. Cover and chill for four hours to one day.
15. When you're ready to enjoy it, arrange the wedges of raspberries and melon balls over the cheesecake.
16. Garnish as desired with fresh oregano and thyme. Slice into wedges to serve.

Servings Provided: 2

Time Required: 1 hour

Macro Counts - Each Serving:

- Calories: 165
- Carbs: 6 g
- Sugar: 3.5 g
- Chol: 12 mg
- Prot.: 32.5 g
- Sodium: 560 mg
- Fat Content: 0.5 g (Saturated: -0- g)
- Net Carbs: 6 g

Ingredients Needed:

- Low fat cottage cheese (8.5 oz.)
- Egg whites (2)
- Vanilla protein powder (1 scoop)
- Stevia (1 tbsp.)
- Vanilla extract (1 tsp.)
- S.F. Strawberry Jell-O (1 serving)
- Water

Preparation Technique:

- Warm the oven to 325° F/163° C.
- Prepare the Jell-O per the package directions and pop it in the freezer.
- Blend the cottage cheese with the egg whites until the consistency is smooth.
- Empty the blended mixture into a mixing container and whisk it with the protein powder, vanilla extract, and stevia.
- Scoop the batter into a small nonstick pan and bake for 25 minutes.
- Extinguish the heat in the oven, leaving the cake in it while it cools down. Once the oven has cooled, remove the cheesecake.
- When the Jell-O is almost set, pour it over the cheesecake.

☐ Let the cake become firm in the fridge for about 10-12 hours before serving.

Servings Provided: 12

Time Required: 25 minutes + chill time

Macro Counts - Each Serving:

- Calories: 237
- Carbs: 27 g
- Sugar: 17 g
- Fiber: 2 g
- Chol: 14 mg
- Prot.: 14 g
- Sodium: 576 mg
- Fat Content: 7 g (Saturated: 4 g)
  D.E:
- Starch: 2
- Fat: 1
- Lean Meat: 1

Ingredients Needed:

- Graham cracker crumbs (.75 cup)
- Unflavored gelatin (1 envelope)
- Water (1 cup - *cold*)
- Melted butter (2 tbsp.)
- Semisweet chocolate (4 oz.)
- F.F. cream cheese (4 pkg. @ 8 oz. each)
- Sugar (.5 cup)
- Sugar substitute (equal to 1 cup sugar)
- Baking cocoa (.25 cup)
- Vanilla extract (2 tsp.)
- Fresh raspberries (2 cups)

Preparation Technique:

1. Crush the cracker crumbs and mix with the butter, pressing it into the base of a greased nine-inch springform pan.
2. Set a timer to bake at 375° Fahrenheit or 191° Celsius until nicely browned (8-10 min.). Wait for a few minutes for it to cool in the pan over a wire rack.
3. Coarsely chop the chocolate. Prepare the filling in a saucepan.
4. Pour the gelatin into chilled water and wait for one minute. Warm it using the low-temperature setting, stirring until gelatin is thoroughly liquified. Mix in the semisweet chocolate, stirring until melted.
5. In another container, combine the sugar substitute with the cream cheese and sugar until smooth. Slowly, mix the chocolate mixture with the coco, beating in the vanilla. Empty the mixture into the crust. Pop it in the fridge until firm (2-3 hrs.).
6. Arrange raspberries on top of the cheesecake. Loosen the edges of the cake from the pan using a knife. Serve as desired.

Chapter 8

Tasty Fruits & Tarts

Fruity Desserts

Servings Provided: 6

Time Required: 1 hour

Macro Counts - Each Serving:

- Calories: 148
- Carbs: 29.7 g
- Sugar: 16.5 g
- Fiber: 3.9 g
- Chol: 5.1 mg
- Protein: 2.7 g
- Sodium: 20.2 mg
- Fat Content: 3 g (Saturated: 1 g)
  D.E.:
- Starch: ½
- Fat: ½
- Fruit: 1
- Other Carbohydrate: ½

Ingredients Needed:

- Regular rolled oats (.5 cup)
- Whole-wheat pastry flour (2 tbsp.)

- ☐ Brown sugar - divided & packed (2 tbsp. + 1 tbsp.)
- ☐ Ground cinnamon (.5 tsp.)
- ☐ Cold butter (1 tbsp.)
- ☐ Golden Delicious apples (3 medium)
- ☐ Fresh lemon juice (1 tbsp.)
- ☐ Water (2 tbsp.)
- ☐ Frozen or low-fat vanilla yogurt (8 oz. container)

Preparation Technique:

1. Warm the oven to reach 350° Fahrenheit or 177 ° Celsius.
2. Combine the oats with the flour, cinnamon, and two tablespoons of brown sugar. Thoroughly stir until combined.
3. Cube and add the butter. Work it in until the mixture begins to form clumps.
4. Core the apples and slice them into thin wedges.
5. Toss the apples with the lemon juice, water, and remaining one tablespoon of brown sugar in a big mixing container. Scoop the apple mixture to a nine-inch pie plate. Sprinkle the oat mixture evenly over the apples.
6. Bake until the topping is nicely browned and the apples are juicy tender (40-45 min.). Serve warm with yogurt if desired.

Servings Provided: 6

Time Required: 15 minutes

Macro Counts - Each Serving:

- ☐ Calories: 97
- ☐ Carbs: 20 g
- ☐ Sugar: 17 g
- ☐ Fiber: 1 g
- ☐ Chol: -0- mg
- ☐ Prot.: 1 g
- ☐ Sodium: 35 mg
- ☐ Fat Content: 2 g (Saturated: -0- g)
  D.E:
- ☐ Starch: ½
- ☐ Fat: ½
- ☐ Fruit: ½

Ingredients Needed:

- ☐ Fresh pineapple (1)
- ☐ Brown sugar (3 tbsp.)
- ☐ Lime juice (1 tbsp.)
- ☐ Honey/agave nectar (1 tbsp.)
- ☐ Olive oil (1 tbsp.)
- ☐ Chili powder (1.5 tsp.)
- ☐ Salt (1 dash)

Preparation Technique:

1. Peel the pineapple, removing any eyes from the fruit. Cut lengthwise into six wedges; remove the core. Mix the rest of the fixings until blended in a mixing container.
2. Brush the pineapple with half of the glaze; reserve the remaining mixture for basting.

3. Cover and grill the pineapple using the medium-temperature setting. Or - broil about four inches from the burner's heat for two to four minutes per side or until lightly browned, occasionally basting with the reserved glaze.

Servings Provided: 5

Time Required: 4 hours 10 minutes

Macro Counts - Each Serving:

- ☐ Calories: 136
- ☐ Carbs: 31 g
- ☐ Sugar: 25 g
- ☐ Fiber: 4 g
- ☐ Sodium: 6 mg
- ☐ Chol: -0- mg
- ☐ Fat Content: 2 g (Saturated: -0- g)
- ☐ Protein: 1 g
  D.E:
- ☐ Starch: 1
- ☐ Fruit: 1

Ingredients Needed:

- ☐ Apples (5 medium)
- ☐ Fresh or frozen cranberries (.33 cup)
- ☐ Chopped walnuts (2 tbsp.)
- ☐ Ground nutmeg (.125 tsp.)
- ☐ Packed brown sugar (.25 cup)
- ☐ Ground cinnamon (.25 tsp.)
- ☐ Optional: Vanilla ice cream or Whipped cream
- ☐ Also Needed: 5-quart slow cooker

Preparation Technique:

1. Thaw and chop the berries.
2. Core the apples, leaving bottoms intact. Peel the top 1/3 of each apple and put it into the cooker.
3. Mix the brown sugar with cinnamon, nutmeg, walnuts, and cranberries. Scoop it over the apples.

4. Securely close the lid and set the setting on low until apples are tender (4-5 hrs.).

5. Garnish and serve as desired.

Servings Provided: 16

Time Required: 35 minutes + cooling time

Macro Counts - Each Serving:

- Calories: 170
- Carbs: 20 g
- Fiber: 1 g
- Sugar: 13 g
- Sodium: 120 mg
- Prot.: 3 g
- Chol: 25 mg
- Fat Content: 9 g (Saturated: 6 g)
  D.E:
- Starch: 1
- Fat: 1 ½
- Fruit: ½

Ingredients Needed:

- Confectioners' sugar (.25 cup)
- A.P. flour (1 cup)
- Cubed cold butter (.5 cup)
- *The Glaze*:
- Lemon juice (1 tsp.)
- Cornstarch (5 tsp.)
- Pineapple juice - unsweetened (1.25 cup)
  The Toppings:
- Reduced-fat cream cheese (8 oz. pkg.)
- Sugar (.33 cup)
- Vanilla extract (1 tsp.)
- Fresh strawberries (2 cups - halved)
- Mandarin oranges - drained (11 oz. can)
- Fresh blueberries (1 cup)

☐ Also Needed: 12-inch pizza pan

Preparation Technique:

1. Warm the oven to 350° Fahrenheit or 177 ° Celsius.
2. Whisk or sift the flour with the confectioners' sugar. Cut/mix in the butter until the mixture is crumbly. Work and press the mixture into an ungreased pan.
3. Bake it until very lightly browned (9-12 min.). Cool it thoroughly on a wire rack.
4. Use a small saucepan to mix glaze fixings until smooth. Wait for it to boil. Simmer and stir until thickened (about 2 min.). Cool slightly.
5. In another container, cream the sugar with the cream cheese and vanilla until it's creamy. Spread it over the crust and top with berries and oranges. Drizzle with the glaze and refrigerate until cold.

Servings Provided: 1

Time Required: 20 minutes

Macro Counts - Each Serving:

- ☐ Calories: 320
- ☐ Carbs: 34.8 g
- ☐ Sugar: 7.7 g
- ☐ Fiber: 11.6 g
- ☐ Chol: 12.5 mg
- ☐ Protein: 29.6 g
- ☐ Sodium: 71.7 mg
- ☐ Fat Content: 8.6 g (Saturated: g)
- ☐ Net Carbs: 23.2

Ingredients Needed:

- ☐ Fresh or frozen raspberries/mixed berries (1 cup/125 g)
- ☐ Stevia (1 tsp.)
- ☐ Vanilla protein powder (1 scoop)
- ☐ Oats (.25 cup/20g)
- ☐ Lemon juice (2 tbsp.)
- ☐ Almonds (10)
- ☐ Also Needed: Small Pyrex oven dish

Preparation Technique:

1. Set the oven temperature at 350° F/177 ° C.
2. Toss the berries into the oven dish and dust with the Stevia over the top.
3. Combine the protein powder with oats and lemon juice. Chop the almonds into small pieces and mix them with the crumble.
4. Spread the crumble over the berries.
5. Set a timer to bake for 15 minutes. Adjust the temperature setting to broil and bake the crumble for another one to two minutes until the top is browned to your liking.
6. Place the pan on the countertop to cool slightly before serving.

Servings Provided: 8

Time Required: 8 ½ hours

Macro Counts - Each Serving:

- 2/3 cup portion:
- Calories: 147
- Carbs: 27 g
- Fiber: 1 g
- Sugar: 14 g
- Chol: 37 mg
- Prot.: 5 g
- Sodium: 35 mg
- Fat Content: 3 g (Saturated: 2 g)
  D.E.:
- Starch: 1
- Fat: ½
- Fruit: ½
- Other Carbohydrate: ½

Ingredients Needed:

- Mangoes - frozen or refrigerated (16 oz.) or (2 medium + more for garnish)
- Light agave syrup (2 tbsp.)
- Almond extract (.25 tsp.)
- Frozen light whipped topping - thawed (1 cup)
- N.F. Greek yogurt - vanilla (1 cup)
- Crisp ladyfingers- Ex. Alessi Biscotti Savoiardi - broken into 1-inch pieces (12)

Preparation Technique:

1. Cube and add half of the mango in a food processor and pulse until it's creamy. Empty the puree into a small bowl. Mix in agave syrup and almond extract.
2. Pulse the remaining mango in the food processor until coarsely chopped. Set aside.

3. Gently fold whipped topping into yogurt in another small bowl. Sprinkle half the ladyfinger pieces into a two-quart shallow baking dish. Spoon half the mango puree and half the yogurt mixture over them. Top with the chopped mango.

4. Layer on the remaining ladyfingers, puree, and yogurt.

5. Gently fold whipped topping into yogurt in another small bowl. Sprinkle half the ladyfinger pieces into the baking dish. Spoon half the mango puree and half the yogurt mixture over them. Top with the chopped mango.

6. Layer on the remaining ladyfingers, puree, and yogurt.

Servings Provided: 4

Time Required: 15 minutes + marinate time

Macro Counts - Each Serving:

- ¾ cup portions:
- Calories: 86
- Carbs: 20 g
- Sugar: 16 g
- Fiber: -0- g
- Chol: -0- mg
- Prot.: 1 g
- Sodium: 7 mg
- Fat Content: -0- g
  D.E:
- Fruit: 1 ½

Ingredients Needed:

- Grated orange zest (1 tbsp.)
- Vanilla extract (1 tsp.)
- Zested lemon (1 tsp.)
- Orange juice (1 cup)
- Sugar (1 tbsp.)
- Lemon juice (1 tbsp.)
  ****
- Medium oranges (4/about 3 cups)
- Optional: Lime zest strips & vanilla yogurt

Preparation Technique:

1. Mix the fixings up to the line (***), stirring until sugar is dissolved.
2. Peel and thinly slice the oranges. Add them to a glass bowl, and add the juice mixture.
3. Refrigerate, covered, until flavors are blended (2-3 hrs.). If desired, top with lime zest strips and serve with yogurt.

Servings Provided: 4

Time Required: 20 minutes + chill time

Macro Counts - Each Serving:

- ☐ Calories: 124
- ☐ Carbs: 29 g
- ☐ Sugar: 21 g
- ☐ Fiber: 3 g
- ☐ Chol: 10 mg
- ☐ Prot.: 2 g
- ☐ Sodium: 67 mg
- ☐ Fat Content: 1 g (Saturated: -0- g)
  D.E.:
- ☐ Starch: 1
- ☐ Fruit: 1

Ingredients Needed:

- ☐ Water (2 tbsp.)
- ☐ Sugar (2 tbsp.)
- ☐ Cornstarch (.5 tsp.)
- ☐ Fresh strawberries - divided (2 cups)
- ☐ Grated lime zest (.5 tsp.)
- ☐ Fresh blueberries (2 cups)
- ☐ Round sponge cakes (2 @ individually-sized)
- ☐ Optional: Whipped topping
- ☐ Also Needed: Wide-mouth half-pint canning jars (4)

Preparation Technique:

1. Use a saucepan to combine the cornstarch with the sugar. Pour in the water. Slice and add one cup of the strawberries and mash the mixture. Wait for it to boil and cook - stirring until thickened (1-2 min.). Transfer the pan to a cool spot and mix in lime zest. Pour it into a small container and pop it into the fridge, covered until chilled.

2. Slice the sponge cakes crosswise into halves. Trim them to fit in the bottoms of the jars.

3. Toss the blueberries and the rest of the strawberries over the cakes. Pour the sauce over the tops and garnish to your liking.

Servings Provided: 1

Time Required: 10 minutes

Macro Counts - Each Serving:

- ☐ Calories: 76
- ☐ Carbs: 12.7 g
- ☐ Sugar: 7.7 g
- ☐ Fiber: 0.7 g
- ☐ Chol: 2 mg
- ☐ Protein: 0.8 g
- ☐ Sodium: 21.1 mg
- ☐ Fat Content: 2.6 g (Saturated: 0.8 g)
  D.E.:
- ☐ Starch: ½
- ☐ Other Carbohydrate: ½

Ingredients Needed:

- ☐ Marshmallow (1)
- ☐ Chocolate-hazelnut spread (.5 tsp.)
- ☐ Ladyfingers (2)
- ☐ Lemon thins (2)
- ☐ Strawberry slices (2)

Preparation Technique:

1. Toast the marshmallow over a fire.
2. Spread the chocolate-hazelnut spread over a lemon thin.
3. Top it off using the marshmallow, strawberry, and the second lemon thin.

Servings Provided: 6

Time Required: 20 minutes

Macro Counts - Each Serving:

- 2/3 cup portions:
- Calories: 101
- Carbs: 26.9 g
- Sugar: 21.5 g
- Fiber: 3.8 g
- Chol: -0- mg
- Prot.: 0.4 g
- Sodium: 2.1 mg
- Fat Content: 0.3 g (Saturated: 0.1 g)
  D.E.:
- Other Carbohydrate: 1
- Fruit: 1

Ingredients Needed:

- Red-skinned cooking apples - ex. Jonathon or Rome (5 medium/about 7 cups)
- Water (.25 cup)
- Cinnamon (.5 tsp.)
- Ground nutmeg(.125 tsp./as desired)
- Honey (2 tbsp.)

Preparation Technique:

1. Remove the core, quarter, and thinly slice the apples.
2. Combine the apple slices with the water in a large skillet. Sprinkle with nutmeg and cinnamon. Once boiling, lower the temperature setting.
3. Place a lid on the pot and simmer until the apples are just tender, stirring once or twice (3 min.).
4. Drizzle with honey and toss to coat.
5. Scoop the serve warm in six individual serving bowls.

Tarts

Servings Provided: 8

Time Required: 35 minutes

Macro Counts - Each Serving:

- ☐ Calories: 190
- ☐ Carbs: 30 g
- ☐ Sugar: 14 g
- ☐ Fiber: 1 g
- ☐ Sodium: 198 mg
- ☐ Prot.: 2 g
- ☐ Chol: 5 mg
- ☐ Fat Content: 7 g (Saturated: 3 g)
  D.E.:
- ☐ Starch: 1 ½
- ☐ Fat: 1
- ☐ Fruit: ½

Ingredients Needed:

- ☐ Refrigerated pie crust (12-inch sheet)
- ☐ Cornstarch (1 tbsp.)
- ☐ Sugar (3 tbsp.)
- ☐ Crystallized ginger (2 tsp.)
- ☐ Egg white (1 large)
- ☐ Water (1 tbsp.)

Preparation Technique:

1. Slice the plums and finely chop the ginger. Cover a baking tray using a sheet of parchment baking paper.
2. Set the oven to 400° Fahrenheit/204° Celsius.
3. Unroll the crust and place it on the prepared tray.

4. Toss the plums with cornstarch and sugar. Place them over the crust to within two inches of its edges and sprinkle with ginger. Fold the crust edge over plums, pleating as you go.

5. Whisk the egg white and water, making an egg wash to brush over the folded crust. Sprinkle with the rest of the sugar.

6. Bake until the crust is nicely browned (18-25 min.). Wait for it to cool in the pan.

7. Once it's cooled, serve as desired.

Servings Provided: 12

Time Required: 40 minutes

Macro Counts - Each Serving:

- ☐ Calories: 199
- ☐ Carbs: 25 g
- ☐ Sugar: 18 g
- ☐ Fiber: 1 g
- ☐ Chol: 36 mg
- ☐ Protein: 4 g
- ☐ Fat Content: 9 g (Saturated: 5 g)
- ☐ Sodium: 112 mg
  D.E.:
- ☐ Starch: 1 ½
- ☐ Fat: 2

Ingredients Needed:

- ☐ Unchilled butter (3 tbsp.)
- ☐ Sugar (.5 cup)
- ☐ A.P. flour (.75 cup)
- ☐ Ground cinnamon (.75 tsp.)
- ☐ Finely chopped walnuts (.33 cup)
  The Filling:
- ☐ Reduced-fat cream cheese (8 oz. pkg.)
- ☐ Sugar - divided (.25 cup + 1 tbsp.)
- ☐ Unchille egg (1 large)
- ☐ Vanilla extract (1 tsp.)
- ☐ Reduced-sugar sliced pears (15 oz. can)
- ☐ Ground cinnamon (.25 tsp.)
- ☐ Also Needed: Nine-inch fluted tart pan & removable bottom.

Preparation Technique:

1. Set the oven to reach 425° F/218° C.
2. Thoroughly drain and thinly slice the pears. Mix the butter with the sugar and cinnamon until crumbly. Mix in the walnuts and flour. Work, pushing the dough mix into bottom and up sides of the pan coated with cooking spray.
3. Make the filling by mixing the cream cheese and sugar (¼ cup) until it's creamy.
4. Whisk in the egg and vanilla. Spread into the crust.
5. Arrange the sliced pears over the top. Mix the cinnamon and the rest of the sugar and sprinkle over the pears.
6. Bake for ten minutes. Adjust the oven's temperature setting to 350° Fahrenheit or 177 ° Celsius.
7. Bake until the filling is set (15 to 20 min.).
8. Cool it for one hour on a wire rack. Pop it into the fridge for a minimum of two hours before serving.

Chapter 9

Brownies & Fudge

Servings Provided: 16

Time Required: 40 minutes

Macro Counts - Each Serving:

- ☐ Calories: 154
- ☐ Carbs: 22 g
- ☐ Sugar: 15 g
- ☐ Fiber: 1 g
- ☐ Chol: 21 mg
- ☐ Prot.: 2 g
- ☐ Sodium: 65 mg
- ☐ Fat Content: 7 g (Saturated: 3 g)
  D.E.:
- ☐ Starch: 1 ½
- ☐ Fat: 1 ½

Ingredients Needed:

- ☐ Unchilled butter - softened (.25 cup)
- ☐ Sugar (.75 cup)
- ☐ Egg (1 large)
- ☐ Baking soda (.5 tsp.)
- ☐ A.P. flour (1 cup)
- ☐ Baking cocoa (1 tbsp.)

- ☐ Ground cinnamon (.5 tsp.)
- ☐ Applesauce (1 cup)
- ☐ The Topping:
- ☐ Chocolate chips (.5 cup)
- ☐ Chopped walnuts/pecans (.5 cup)
- ☐ Sugar (1 tbsp.)
- ☐ Needed: Eight-inch square baking pan

Preparation Technique:

1. Combine the butter with the sugar in a big mixing container. Beat and mix in the egg.
2. Sift to combine the cocoa with the baking soda, flour, and cinnamon. Slowly add and mix into the creamed mixture. Fold in the applesauce.
3. Spritz the baking tray using a portion of cooking oil spray and add the mix.
4. Toss and sprinkle the topping fixings over the batter.
5. Bake at 350° Fahrenheit or 177 ° Celsius until done (25 min.). Cool the brownies over a wire rack before cutting them into 16 squares.

Servings Provided: 12

Time Required: 45 minutes

Macro Counts - Each Serving:

- ☐ Calories: 172
- ☐ Carbs: 23 g
- ☐ Sugar: 18 g
- ☐ Chol: 36 mg
- ☐ Prot.: 4 g
- ☐ Sodium: 145 mg
- ☐ Fat Content: 8 g (Saturated: 5 g)
  D.E.:
- ☐ Starch: 1 ½
- ☐ Fat: 1 ½ fat

Ingredients Needed:

- ☐ Eggs - divided (3 large)
- ☐ Unchilled reduced-fat butter (6 tbsp.)
- ☐ Sugar - divided (1 cup)
- ☐ Baking cocoa (.25 cup)
- ☐ Vanilla extract (3 tsp.)
- ☐ A.P. flour (.5 cup)
- ☐ Reduced-fat cream cheese (8 oz. pkg.)
- ☐ Needed: 9-inch square baking pan

Preparation Technique:

1. Warm the oven to reach 350° F/177 ° C.
2. Separate two eggs (tossing the yolks), putting each white in a separate bowl, and place it to the side for now.
3. Combine and mix 3/4 cup sugar with the butter until crumbly. Whisk and mix in one egg white, the remaining whole egg, and vanilla - mixing until it's thoroughly combined.

4. Whisk or sift the flour and cocoa, slowly adding it to the egg mixture until blended. Empty it into the baking pan coated with cooking spray; set aside.

5. Mix the cream cheese with the rest of the sugar until smooth. Fold in the second egg white. Drop by rounded tablespoonfuls over the batter, cutting through the batter with a knife to swirl.

6. Bake until set and edges pull away from the pan's sides (25-30 min.). Cool on a wire rack and serve.

Servings Provided: 40 squares

Time Required: 5 minutes + chill time 2 hours

Macro Counts - Each Serving:

- ☐ Calories: 122
- ☐ Carbs: 5.85 g
- ☐ Sugar: 2.97 g
- ☐ Fiber: 2.28g
- ☐ Prot.: 1.325 g
- ☐ Sodium: mg
- ☐ Fat Content: 11 g (Saturated: 8.8 g)

Ingredients Needed:

- ☐ Coconut butter (1.5 cups)
- ☐ Full-fat coconut milk (13.66 fl. oz. can)
- ☐ Bittersweet chocolate chips (10 oz.)
- ☐ Optional Topping: Flaked/coarse sea salt
- ☐ Also Suggested: 8 by 8-inch baking pan

Preparation Technique:

1. Line the baking pan with a layer of foil or waxed paper.
2. Melt the coconut butter in a saucepan using the low-temperature setting.
3. Mix in the chips and milk. Let the mixture simmer, frequently stirring until the chocolate has melted.
4. Empty the batter into the prepared baking pan. Drizzle with sea salt and pop it into the fridge until it's set (2 hrs.). Slice and serve.

Servings Provided: 16

Time Required: 40 minutes

Macro Counts - Each Serving:

- ☐ Calories: 150
- ☐ Carbs: 19 g
- ☐ Sugar: 13 g
- ☐ Chol: 27 mg
- ☐ Prot.: 2 g
- ☐ Sodium: 68 mg
- ☐ Fat Content: 8 g (Saturated: 1 g)
  D.E.:
- ☐ Starch: 1
- ☐ Fat: 1 ½

Ingredients Needed:

- ☐ Mashed potatoes (.75 cup)
- ☐ Sugar (.5 cup)
- ☐ Brown sugar - tightly packed (.5 cup)
- ☐ Eggs (2 large)
- ☐ Canola oil (.5 cup)
- ☐ Vanilla extract (1 tsp.)
- ☐ A.P. flour (.5 cup)
- ☐ Salt (.125 tsp.)
- ☐ Cocoa powder (.33 cup)
- ☐ Baking powder (.5 tsp.)
- ☐ Optional: Chopped pecans (.5 cup)
- ☐ Confectioners' sugar
- ☐ Suggested: 9-inch square baking tray

Preparation Technique:

1. Combine the mashed potatoes with the sugars, eggs, oil, and vanilla.

2. Sift the flour with the salt, cocoa, and baking powder; slowly adding the mixture into the potato mixture. Fold in the pecans and pour into a greased pan.
3. Bake at 350° Fahrenheit or 177 ° Celsius until a toothpick inserted in the center comes out clean (for 23-27 min.). Put the pan on a wire rack to cool.
4. Sprinkle using confectioners' sugar. Cut into 16 bars. Serve as desired.

Chapter 10

Cookie Favorites

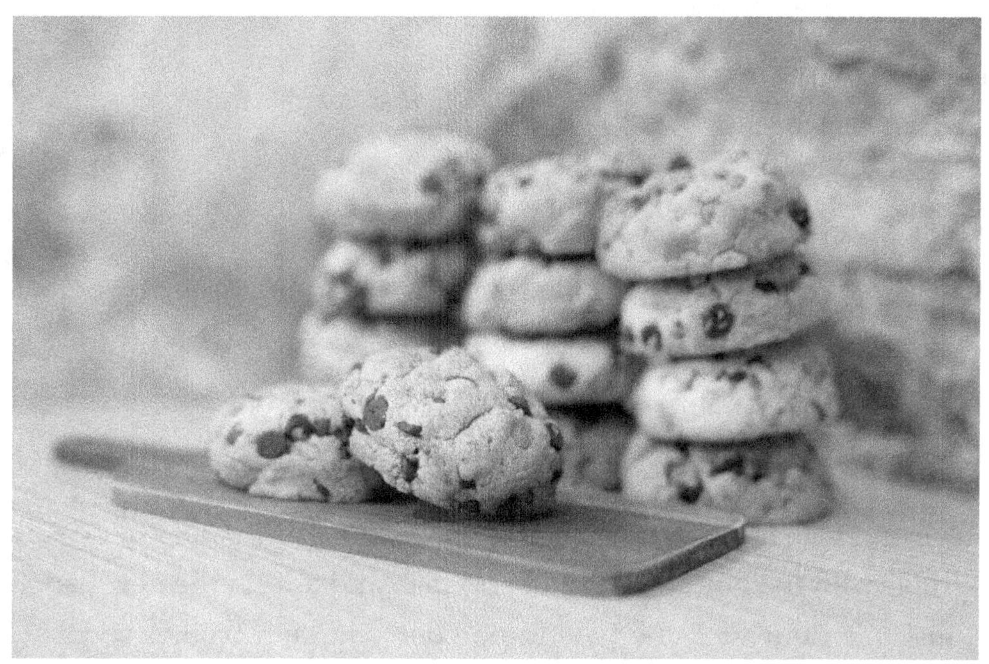

Servings Provided: 3 d0zen

Time Required: 35 minutes

Macro Counts - Each Serving:

- ☐ Calories: 69
- ☐ Carbs: 10 g
- ☐ Sugar: 6 g
- ☐ Fiber: -0- g
- ☐ Sodium: 50 mg
- ☐ Protein: 1 g
- ☐ Chol: 10 mg

- ☐ Fat Content: 3 g (Saturated: 2 g)
  D.E.:
- ☐ Starch: ½
- ☐ Fat: ½

Ingredients Needed:

- ☐ Unchilled butter (.33 cup)
- ☐ Sugar (.5 cup)
- ☐ Unchilled egg (1 large)
- ☐ Vanilla extract (.5 tsp.)
- ☐ Mashed ripe banana (.5 cup)
- ☐ A.P. flour (1.25 cups)
- ☐ Bak. powder (1 tsp.)
- ☐ Salt (.25 tsp.)
- ☐ Bak. soda (.125 tsp.)
- ☐ Semisweet chocolate chips (1 cup)

Preparation Technique:

- ☐ Mix the sugar with the butter until fluffy. Whisk and add in the egg, banana, and vanilla. Sift or whisk the flour with the baking powder, salt, and baking soda, slowly adding it into the creamed mixture. Fold in the chocolate chips.
- ☐ Drop by tablespoonfuls about two inches apart onto baking trays coated with cooking oil spray.
- ☐ Bake at 350° Fahrenheit/177 ° Celsius until the edges are browned (13-16 min.). Transfer the pans to wire racks to cool.
- ☐ Serve and enjoy them anytime.

Servings Provided: 7 dozen

Time Required: 25 minutes

Macro Counts - Each Serving:

- ☐ Calories: 50
- ☐ Carbs: 6 g
- ☐ Sugar: 3 g
- ☐ Protein: 1 g
- ☐ Chol: 5 mg
- ☐ Sodium: 24 mg
- ☐ Fat Content: 2 g (Saturated: -0- g)
  D.E.:
- ☐ Starch: ½
- ☐ Fat: ½

Ingredients Needed:

- ☐ Shortening (.66 cup)
- ☐ Brown sugar - tightly packed (1 cup)
- ☐ Unchilled large eggs (2)
- ☐ Buttermilk (.5 cup)
- ☐ Vanilla extract (1 tsp.)
- ☐ A.P. flour (2 cups)
- ☐ Salt (.5 tsp.)
- ☐ Bak. soda (.25 tsp.)
- ☐ Ground cloves (.25 tsp.)
- ☐ Bak. powder (.25 tsp.)
- ☐ Ground nutmeg (.25 tsp.)
- ☐ Cinnamon (1 tsp.)
- ☐ Shredded carrots (1 cup)
- ☐ Oats - Quick-cooking type (2 cups)
- ☐ Pecans (.5 cup)

Preparation Technique:

1. Combine the shortening with the brown sugar until light and fluffy (5-7 min.). Whisk and mix in the eggs with the buttermilk and vanilla. Whisk the flour with the salt, baking powder, cinnamon, cloves, baking soda, and nutmeg. Slowly mix it into the creamed mixture.
2. Chop and mix in the pecans, carrots, and oats.
3. Scoop and drop the dough by rounded teaspoonfuls onto ungreased baking sheets (2 in. apart).
4. Set the timer to bake at 375° Fahrenheit or 191° Celsius until lightly browned (6-8 min.). Place the pans onto wire racks to cool.
5. You have a freezer option. Scoop them by teaspoonfuls onto parchment-lined baking sheets. Freeze until firm. Transfer the cookie dough balls to zipper-type bags or other freezer containers; seal tightly and freeze for up to three months. To bake, place the frozen dough two inches apart on ungreased baking sheets.
6. Bake at 375° Fahrenheit or 191° Celsius until browned for 10-15 minutes (since the dough is chilled). Transfer them onto wire racks to cool.

Servings Provided: 36

Time Required: 50 minutes

Macro Counts - Each Serving:

- Calories: 98
- Carbs: 14 g
- Fiber: 1 g
- Sugar: 8 g
- Chol: 12 mg
- Prot.: 2 g
- Fat Content: 4 g (Saturated: 2 g)
- Sodium: 115 mg
  D.E.:
- Starch: ½
- Fat: 1/2
- Other Carbohydrate: ½

Ingredients Needed:

- Unchilled butter (.5 cup)
- Brown sugar (1 cup - packed)
- Ground cinnamon (1 tsp.)
- Salt (.25 tsp.)
- Bak. soda (2 tsp.)
- Ground ginger (1 tsp.)
- Egg (1)
- Unsweetened applesauce (.25 cup)
- Vanilla (1 tsp.)
- Whole wheat flour (2 cups)
- Carrots, finely shredded (1 cup/2 medium)
- Raisins (.75 cup)
- Finely chopped walnuts (.75 cup)

Preparation Technique:

1. Warm the oven to reach 375° F/191° C.
2. Combine the butter using an electric mixer using the medium speed setting for ½ minute.
3. Measure and mix in the baking soda, brown sugar, cinnamon, ginger, and salt, thoroughly mixing until combined.
4. Mix in the egg, applesauce, and vanilla. Fold in any remaining flour, raisins, carrots, and walnuts - just until combined.
5. Drop by slightly rounded teaspoons two inches apart onto ungreased baking trays.
6. Bake until the edges are firm (8-9 min.).
7. Place the cookies onto a wire rack to thoroughly cool.

Servings Provided: 40

Time Required: 45 minutes

Macro Counts - Each Serving:

- ☐ Calories: 78
- ☐ Fiber: 1 g
- ☐ Carbs: 10 g
- ☐ Chol: 3 mg
- ☐ Prot.: 2 g
- ☐ Sodium: 47 mg
- ☐ Fat Content: 4 g (Saturated: 2 g)
  D.E.:
- ☐ Fat: ½
- ☐ Carb Choices: ½
- ☐ Other Carb: ½

Ingredients Needed:

- ☐ Boiling water (.5 cup)
- ☐ Raisins (1 cup)
- ☐ Peanut butter (.5 cup)
- ☐ Unchilled butter (.25 cup)
- ☐ Sugar (.5 cup)
- ☐ Baking soda (.5 tsp.)
- ☐ Refrigerated or frozen egg product - thawed (.5 cup)
- ☐ Ground cinnamon (1 tsp.)
- ☐ Vanilla (1 tsp.)
- ☐ A.P. flour (.5 cup)
- ☐ Regular rolled oats (1.25 cups)
- ☐ Chocolate chunks - semi-sweet (1 cup)

Preparation Technique:

1. Warm the oven temperature to reach 350° Fahrenheit/177 ° Celsius.

2. Cover cookie sheets with parchment baking paper, if desired.
3. Toss the raisins and boiling water in a mixing dish and set it aside.
4. Cream the peanut butter with the butter or beat with an electric mixer using the medium-speed setting for ½ minute.
5. Add the cinnamon, sugar substitute, baking soda, egg product, and vanilla. Blend until incorporated.
6. Mix in the flour, and lastly, the oats.
7. Drain the raisins and combine with the chocolate pieces, adding them into the oat mixture.
8. Drop the batter by rounded teaspoons onto the prepared baking trays.
9. Bake them until lightly browned (10 min.).
10. Place the pans onto wire racks to cool.

Servings Provided: 12

Time Required: 40 minutes

Macro Counts - Each Serving:

- Calories: 156
- Carbs: 5.4 g
- Fiber: 2.3 g
- Sugar: 1.1 g
- Chol: -0- mg
- Prot.: 4.2 g
- Sodium: 94.1 mg
- Fat Content: 14.1 g (Saturated: 4.4 g)
- Net Carbs: 3.1 g

Ingredients Needed:

- Almond flour (2 cups)
- Bak. powder (.5 tsp.)
- Sea salt (.5 tsp.)
- Flaxseed powder (1 tbsp.)
- Water (3 tbsp.)
- Unsweetened pumpkin puree (.5 cup)
- Coconut oil (.25 cup)
- Coconut oil (1 tsp./as needed)
- Vanilla extract (1 tsp.)
- Brown erythritol (.5 cup)
- Ground cinnamon (2 tsp.)
- To Garnish: Brown erythritol (4 tsp.)

Preparation Technique:

1. Warm the oven at 350° Fahrenheit/177 ° Celsius.
2. Prepare a cookie tray with a layer of parchment baking paper.
3. Sift the almond flour with the salt and baking powder in a mixing container.

4. Prepare a "flax egg" by mixing one tablespoon of flax powder and three tablespoons of water in a mixing cup or another container. Wait for five minutes. (Use one egg if not vegan.)

5. Add the flax egg with the pumpkin puree, melted coconut oil, and vanilla extract into a mixing container, whisking until smooth.

6. Add the erythritol to the wet fixings. Stir until well-combined, and most of the sweetener granules are liquified.

7. Combine the wet fixings to the almond flour mixture until the dough sticks together. (Add small amounts of almond flour if it's too sticky).

8. Oil your hands and roll out the dough (2 tbsp. at a time) into 12 balls and place on the baking sheet. Use a fork to press each ball down crosswise until they're about ½-inch thick.

9. Bake until they're just starting to brown and turn golden (15-20 min.).

10. Transfer the tray to the countertop and sprinkle with cinnamon and brown erythritol while warm.

11. Cool them on the cookie tray for 20 minutes. Gently move them onto a wire cooling rack to finish cooling to serve.

Servings Provided: 2.5 dozen

Time Required: 30 minutes + chill time

Macro Counts - Each Serving:

- ☐ Calories: 77
- ☐ Carbs: 14 g
- ☐ Sugar: 7 g
- ☐ Fiber: 1 g
- ☐ Chol: 7 mg
- ☐ Prot.: 1 g
- ☐ Sodium: 106 mg
- ☐ Fat Content: 2 g (Saturated: -0- g)
  D.E.:
- ☐ Starch: 1

Ingredients Needed:

- ☐ Canola oil (.25 cup)
- ☐ Egg (1 large)
- ☐ Sugar (.66 cup)
- ☐ Molasses (.33 cup)
- ☐ Ground cloves (.25 tsp.)
- ☐ White whole wheat flour (2 cups)
- ☐ Bak. soda (1.5 tsp.)
- ☐ Cinnamon (1 tsp.)
- ☐ Ground ginger (.25 tsp.)
- ☐ Salt (.5 tsp.)
- ☐ Confectioners' sugar (1 tbsp.)

Preparation Technique:

1. Mix the sugar with the oil until blended. Whisk and mix in the egg and molasses.
2. Whisk the flour with the salt, cloves, baking soda, ginger, and cinnamon. Mix it into the sugar mixture.

3. Cover the container and put it into the refrigerator to chill for a minimum of two hours.

4. Warm the oven temperature to reach 350° F/177 ° C.

5. Shape the dough into one-inch balls and roll them in confectioners' sugar.

6. Arrange them about two inches apart onto baking trays coated with cooking spray.

7. Fatten them slightly to bake for seven to nine minutes or until they're firm. Transfer the cookies to wire racks to cool. Serve as desired.

Servings Provided: 6 dozen

Time Required: 45 minutes

Macro Counts - Each Serving:

- Calories: 56
- Carbs: 11 g
- Sugar: 6 g
- Fiber: 1 g
- Chol: 5 mg
- Prot.: 1 g
- Sodium: 40 mg
- Fat Content: 1 g (Saturated: 1 g)
  D.E.:
- Starch: 1

Ingredients Needed:

- Hot water (2 tbsp.)
- Ground flaxseed (1 tbsp.)
- Pitted dried plums (1 cup)
- Dates (1 cup)
- Raisins (.5 cup)
- Unchilled butter (.o.33 cup)
- Brown sugar (.75 cup - packed tight)
- Egg (1 large)
- Vanilla extract (2 tsp.)
- Unsweetened applesauce (.5 cup)
- Maple syrup (.25 cup)
- Grated orange zest (1 tbsp.)
- Oats - quick-cooking (3 cups)
- A.P. flour (1 cup)
- Baking soda (1 tsp.)
- Whole wheat flour (.5 cup)

- ☐ Ground nutmeg & cloves (.25 tsp. each)
- ☐ Salt (.5 tsp.)
- ☐ Cinnamon (1 tsp.)

Preparation Technique:

1. Combine water and flaxseed. Chop the dates and plums.
2. In another container, combine the plums, dates, and raisins. Pour in boiling water. Let the flaxseed and plum mixtures stand for ten minutes.
3. Meanwhile, combine the brown sugar with the butter until light and fluffy.
4. Mix in the whisked egg and vanilla. Beat in the applesauce, maple syrup, and orange zest. Combine the oats with both flours, salt, baking soda, cinnamon, nutmeg, and cloves. Slowly add to the creamed mixture. Drain the plum mixture; stir the plum and flaxseed into the dough.
5. Drop by rounded teaspoonfuls onto lightly greased baking trays (two inches apart). Bake at 350° Fahrenheit or 177 ° Celsius until set (8-11 min.).
6. Cool the cookies for about ten minutes. Remove them from the pans to wire racks.

Servings Provided: 24

Time Required: 20 minutes

Macro Counts - Each Serving:

- Calories: 67
- Carbs: 8 g
- Fiber: 1 g
- Sugar: 5 g
- Chol: 9 mg
- Prot.: 2 g
- Sodium: 57 mg
- Fat Content: 3 g (Saturated: 1 g)
  D.E.:
- Starch: ½
- Fat: ½

Ingredients Needed:

- Peanut butter - chunky-style (.5 cup)
- Brown sugar - packed (.5 cup)
- Egg (1 large)
- Quick-cooking oats (1.25 cups)
- Baking soda (.5 tsp.)

Preparation Technique:

1. Warm the oven to reach 350° F/177 ° C. Grease baking trays.
2. Combine the brown sugar and peanut butter, mixing until fluffy.
3. Whisk and mix in the egg. Fold in the oats and baking soda to the creamed mixture.
4. Thoroughly combine and drop by tablespoonfuls two inches apart onto the prepared cookie trays.
5. Flatten each one slightly. Bake for six to eight minutes and cool over wire racks. Store them in a cookie jar.

Servings Provided: 12

Time Required: 1 hour

Macro Counts - Each Serving:

- Based on 12 cookies:
- Calories: 140
- Carbs: 4 g
- Fiber: 1.2 g
- Chol: 15.4 mg
- Protein: 5.8 g
- Sodium: 134.3 mg
- Fat Content: 10.4 g (Sat. Fat: 2.1 g)
- Net Carbs: 2.8 g

Ingredients Needed:

- Peanut butter - smooth with no-added-sugar (1 cup/250 g)
- Egg (1 large)
- Erythritol (.66 or 2/3 cup/135 g)
- Baking soda (.5 tsp.)
- Vanilla essence (.5 tsp.)
- Suggested: Nutribullet or another high-power blender

Preparation Technique:

1. Warm the oven to 350° Fahrenheit/177 ° Celsius.
2. Line a baking tray using a layer of parchment baking paper. Set aside.
3. Pulse the erythritol in a blender until it's powdered. Place it to the side for now. (If you are using a low-carb confectioner's sweetener, you can omit this step).
4. Toss each of the fixings into a mixing container, whisking until a glossy dough is created.
5. Make the balls by rolling about two tablespoons of dough between your palms to form a ball. Put it on the prepared tray. Continue the process until all of the dough has been used (1 dozen cookies)
6. Flatten the cookies using a fork to create a criss-cross pattern across the tops.

7. Bake the cookies for 11-15 minutes.

8. Transfer them to the countertop to cool for ½ hour on the cookie sheet. At that point, transfer the cookies onto a cooling rack for another 15 minutes to ensure they are cooled before storing.

Servings Provided: 2.5 dozen

Time Required: ½ hour + cooling time

Macro Counts - Each Serving:

- Calories: 102
- Carbs: 11 g
- Sugar: 10 g
- Fiber: 1 g
- Prot.: 2 g
- Sodium: 43 mg
- Chol: 7 mg
- Fat Content: 6 g (Saturated: 2 g)

Ingredients Needed:

- Peanut butter (1 cup)
- Unchilled egg (1 large)
- Sugar (1 cup)
- Vanilla extract (1 tsp.)
- Milk chocolate kisses (30)

Preparation Technique:

1. Warm the oven to reach 350° Fahrenheit/177 ° Celsius.
2. Cream the sugar with the peanut butter until it's fluffy and light. Whisk the vanilla and egg, mixing it into the batter.
3. Roll the mixture into 1.25-inch balls. Arrange them two inches apart onto ungreased cookie trays. Bake until tops are slightly cracked (10-13 min.).
4. Promptly push one of the chocolate kisses into the center of each cookie.
5. Cool the cookies for about five minutes before removing them from the pans to wire racks.

Servings Provided: 24

Time Required: 25 minutes

Macro Counts - Each Serving:

- Calories: 92
- Carbs: 15 g
- Fiber: Trace amounts
- Sodium: 49 mg
- Protein: 1 g
- Chol: 14 mg
- Fat Content: 3 g (Saturated: 1 g)
  D.E.:
- Starch: 1
- Fat: ½

Ingredients Needed:

- Unchilled butter (.25 cup)
- Sugar (.5 cup)
- Brown sugar - packed (.5 cup)
- Canola oil (2 tbsp.)
- Egg (1)
- Vanilla extract (.25 tsp.)
- A.P. flour (1.5 cups)
- Salt (.25 tsp.)
- Baking soda (.125 tsp.)
- Variety Options:
- Yellow and red food coloring
- Beaten egg white
- Popsicle or lollipop sticks

Preparation Technique:

1. Beat the butter with both types of sugars until crumbly (2 min.). Whisk and mix in the egg, oil, and vanilla. Whisk the flour with the salt and baking soda. Slowly add to the mixture.
2. Lightly flour a work surface and divide the dough in half.
3. Roll one piece of the dough into 1/4-inch thickness.
4. Cut with a floured three-inch ghost-shaped (or your favorite) cookie cutter. Arrange the cookies one inch apart on baking sheets coated with cooking spray. Repeat until all of the dough is used.
5. Bake at 350° Fahrenheit or 177 ° Celsius until set (5-6 min.). Cool the cookies for one minute before removing from the pans to wire racks.
6. Decorate as desired.

Servings Provided: 5 dozen

Time Required: 1 hour + standing time

Macro Counts - Each Serving:

- Calories: 10
- Carbs: 2 g
- Sugar: 2 g
- Sodium: 5 mg
- Fat Content: -0- g
  D.E.:
- **Free Food**: 1

Ingredients Needed:

- Egg whites (3 large)
- Clear/regular vanilla extract (1.5 tsp.)
- Salt (1 dash)
- Cream of tartar (.25 tsp.)
- Sugar (2/3 cup)
- Useful: Electric mixer

Preparation Technique:

1. Separate and add the egg whites in a small cup and wait for ½ hour until they are at room temperature.
2. Set the oven temperature to 250° F/121° C.
3. Whisk the salt, vanilla, and cream of tartar into the egg whites, beating using the medium-speed setting until foamy.
4. Slowly mix in the sugar (1 tbsp. @ a time), mixing using the high setting after each addition until the sugar is liquified. Continue to beat it to make stiff glossy peaks (7 min.).
5. Use a pastry bag or cut a small hole in the corner of a "food-safe" plastic bag. Insert a #32-star tip. Transfer the meringue into the bag and pipe 1.25-inch-diameter cookies - two inches apart onto parchment-lined baking sheets.

6. Bake until firm to the touch (40-45 min.).

7. Turn the power off to the oven. Leave the meringues in the warm oven for one hour (oven door closed). Transfer them from the oven and thoroughly cool on the baking trays.

8. Transfer the meringues from the paper and store them in an airtight container at room temperature.

Chapter 11

Snack Bars

Servings Provided: 4 dozen

Time Required: 35 minutes + cool time

Macro Counts - Each Serving:

- ☐ Calories: 68
- ☐ Carbs: 11 g
- ☐ Fiber: -0- g
- ☐ Sugar: 8 g
- ☐ Chol: 7 mg
- ☐ Prot.: 1 g
- ☐ Sodium: 55 mg
- ☐ Fat Content: 2 g (Saturated: 1 g)
  D.E.:
- ☐ Starch: 1
- ☐ Fat: ½

Ingredients Needed:

- ☐ Unchilled butter (.25 cup)
- ☐ Brown sugar - packed (1 cup)
- ☐ Brewed espresso (.5 cup)
- ☐ Egg (1 large)
- ☐ Self-rising flour (1.5 cups)
- ☐ Chopped slivered almonds - toasted (.75 cup)

- ☐ Ground cinnamon (.5 tsp.)
- ☐ The Glaze:
- ☐ Confectioners' sugar (1.5 cups)
- ☐ Water (3 tbsp.)
- ☐ Almond extract (.75 tsp.)
- ☐ Slivered almonds - toasted (.25 cup)
- ☐ Needed: 15x10x1-in. baking pan

Preparation Technique:

1. Mix the butter with the brown sugar and espresso until blended. Whisk and mix in the egg. Whisk the flour with the cinnamon, slowly adding it to the creamed mixture. Chop and stir in the almonds.
2. Spread them onto a greased baking pan. Bake at 350° Fahrenheit or 177 ° Celsius until lightly browned (18-22 min.).
3. In another mixing container, combine the water with the confectioners' sugar and extract until creamy smooth.
4. Spread the mixture over warm bars with a sprinkle with slivered almonds. Cool on a wire rack.
5. Slice them into bars to serve.

Servings Provided: 20

Time Required: 3 hours

Macro Counts - Each Serving:

- Calories: 141
- Carbs: 13.5 g
- Sugar: 7.8 g
- Fiber: 0.6 g
- Chol: 22.9 mg
- Prot.: 4.3 g
- Sodium: 116.2 mg
- Fat Content: 8 g (Saturated: 4.4 g)
  D.E.:
- Fat: 1 ½
- Other Carbohydrate: 1

Ingredients Needed:

- Packed brown sugar (3 tbsp.)
- Almonds - finely chopped (2 tbsp.)
- A.P. flour (.66 cup)
- Rolled oats - quick-cooking (.66 cup)
- Butter (.25 cup)
- Reduced-fat cream cheese - Neufchatel (2 - 8 oz. pkg.)
- Granulated sugar (1/3 cup)
- Vanilla (2 tsp.)
- Almond extract (.25 tsp.)
- Refrigerated/frozen egg product, thawed,(1 cup) or Eggs (4)
- Dried cherries (1/3 cup)
- Optional: F.F. frozen whipped dessert topping (10 tbsp.)
- Optional: Sliced almonds (2 tbsp.)
- Suggested: 8x8x2-inch baking pan

Preparation Technique:

1. Set the oven temperature at 350° F/177 ° C.
2. Thaw the topping.
3. Lightly grease the baking tray or cover it using a foil layer, extending it up and over the edges of the pan. Place it to the side for now.
4. Combine the flour with brown sugar, almonds, and oats.
5. Work or cut in the butter using a pastry blender until it is a bunch of coarse crumbs. Use your hands and push the crumbs into the bottom of the pan.
6. Set a timer to bake for 12 minutes.
7. Beat the cream cheese with the vanilla extract, granulated sugar, and almond extract using an electric mixer on the medium speed setting until it's 'fluffy' and light. Slowly mix in the egg, combining it on the low-speed setting - just until incorporated.
8. Finely chop and stir in the cherries. Spread the cream cheese mixture over the partially baked crust.
9. Bake until the cream cheese layer is set (25-35 min.). Thoroughly cool in the pan on a wire rack. Place a layer of plastic wrap over them and chill for two to 24 hours before serving.
10. Slice them into bars to serve, adding dessert topping or almonds to your liking.
11. Store them in the fridge to keep them fresh.

Servings Provided: 24

Time Required: 50 minutes

Macro Counts - Each Serving:

- Calories: 197
- Carbs: 29 g
- Sugar: 19 g
- Fiber: 2 g
- Chol: 40 mg
- Prot.: 4 g
- Sodium: 157 mg
- Fat Content: 8 g (Saturated: 5 g)
  D.E.:
- Starch: 2
- Fat: 1

Ingredients Needed:

- Butter - cubed (1/3 cup)
- Unsweetened chocolate (1.5 oz.)
- Boiling water (.5 cup)
- Instant coffee granules (1 tbsp.)
- Canned pumpkin (1 cup)
- Eggs - whisked (2 large)
- Sugar (1.5 cups)
- A.P. flour (2 cups)
- Baking soda (.75 tsp.)
- Salt (.5 tsp.)
- The Batter:
- Reduced-fat cream cheese (8 oz. pkg.)
- Canned pumpkin (.5 cup)
- Vanilla extract (1 tsp.)
- Sugar (.25 cup)

☐ Ground cloves (.125 tsp.)

☐ Cinnamon (.75 tsp.)

☐ Ground ginger (.75 tsp.)

☐ Egg - lightly beaten (1 large)

☐ Semisweet chocolate chips (1 cup)

☐ Needed: 15x10x1-inch baking pan

Preparation Technique:

1. Coarsely chop the chocolate.

2. Melt the butter with the chocolate in the microwave, stirring until smooth. Cool slightly.

3. Use a big mixing container, liquify the coffee in water, and mix in the eggs, pumpkin, and chocolate mixture.

4. Whisk the flour with the sugar, baking soda, and salt. Slowly add it to the chocolate mixture. Transfer to the baking pan coated with cooking oil spray.

5. Prepare the cheesecake batter in a mixing container.

6. Combine and mix the pumpkin with the cream cheese until smooth.

7. Fold in the vanilla, sugar, and spices. Whisk and add the egg, beating using the low-speed setting until barely incorporated.

8. Spoon the mixture over the chocolate batter. Swirl the mixture using a knife to mix the cheesecake portion. Sprinkle with chocolate chips.

9. Bake at 350° Fahrenheit or 177 ° Celsius until a toothpick inserted in the center comes out with moist crumbs (20-25 min.). Cool on a wire rack.

10. Cut into bars and refrigerate any leftovers.

Servings Provided: 24

Time Required: ½ hour

Macro Counts - Each Serving:

- Calories: 145
- Carbs: 13 g
- Fiber: 1 g
- Sugar: 8 g
- Chol: 8 mg
- Prot.: 7 g
- Sodium: 203 mg
- Fat Content: g (Saturated: g)
  D.E.:
- Starch: 1
- Fat: 1
- Fruit: 1
- Lean Meat: 1

Ingredients Needed:

- Nonstick cooking spray (as needed)
- Rolled oats - regular cut (.5 cup)
- Whole wheat flour (.5 cup)
- Brown sugar - tightly packed (.25 cup)
- Butter - melted (.25 cup)
- Unchilled - F.F. cream cheese (2 - 8 oz. pkg.)
- Creamy peanut butter (.75 cup)
- Granulated sugar (.33 cup)
- Refrigerated/frozen egg product - thawed (.75 cup)
- F.F. milk (.25 cup + 2 tbsp.)
- Vanilla (1 tsp.)
- Semisweet chocolate - chopped (2 oz.)
- Chopped peanuts (3 tbsp.)

- ☐ Cooking oil spray (as needed)
- ☐ Needed: 13x9x2-inch baking pan

Preparation Technique:

1. Warm the oven to reach 350° F/177 ° C.
2. Spritz the pan using a portion of the oil spray.
3. Measure and toss the oats into a blender/food processor. Securely close the lid and pulse until they are coarsely ground.
4. Toss the ground oats with the brown sugar, flour, and melted butter. Evenly press it into the base of the baking tray.
5. Mix the granulated sugar with the cream cheese and peanut butter, using an electric mixer until combined (medium-speed setting). Pour in ¼ cup of milk, vanilla, and egg substitute. Mix it using the low-speed setting - just until combined.
6. Empty the filling into the prepared crust. Set a timer and bake until set in the center (25 min.).
7. Cool the bars in the pan for ½ hour. Put a layer of foil over the top of the pan. Pop it into the fridge for a minimum of four hours or up to 24 hours.
8. Use a heavy saucepan to melt the chocolate using the low-temperature setting until melted. Transfer the pan to a cool spot and mix in enough milk (2-3 tbsp.) to make it a drizzling consistency.
9. Empty the melted chocolate into a small resealable plastic bag. Seal the bag and snip off a small corner from the bag. Pipe the chocolate over the cheesecake. Sprinkle with chopped peanuts and cover with plastic wrap to cool. Serve when it's set.

Servings Provided: 16

Time Required: 50 minutes + chill time

Macro Counts - Each Serving:

- Calories: 117
- Carbs: 13 g
- Fiber: -0- g
- Sugar: 9 g
- Chol: 31 mg
- Prot.: 3 g
- Sodium: 135 mg
- Fat Content: 6 g (Saturated:4 g)
  D.E.:
- Fat: 1
- Starch: 1

Ingredients Needed:

- Graham cracker crumbs (1 cup)
- Melted butter - reduced-fat (2 tbsp.)
- Sugar (2 tbsp.)
- The Filling:
- R.F. cream cheese (11 oz.)
- R.F. sour cream (.33 cup)
- Sugar (.33 cup)
- A.P. flour (2 tsp.)
- Vanilla extract (.5 tsp.)
- Egg (1 large)
- Brown sugar (1 tbsp.)
- Pumpkin from a can (.5 cup)
- Also Suggested: 9-inch baking dish

Preparation Technique:

1. Toss the sugar with the cracker crumbs. Add in the butter. Press onto the bottom of the dish coated with a spritz of cooking oil spray.
2. Bake at 325° Fahrenheit or 163° Celsius until set (6-10 min.). Remove and place them onto a rack to cool.
3. Prepare the filling in a big mixing container. Mix the sour cream with the cream cheese, flour, sugar, and vanilla until it's creamy smooth. Whisk and mix in the egg, beating on the low setting - just until combined.
4. Remove 3/4 cup of the batter to a mixing container, and fold in brown sugar and pumpkin until thoroughly mixed.
5. Pour plain batter over the crust. Next, spread pumpkin batter over plain batter.
6. Bake at 325° Fahrenheit or 163° Celsius until the center is almost set (20-25 min.).
7. Next, wait for it to cool for one hour on a wire rack.
8. Place a layer of foil or plastic wrap over the bars and pop the pan into the fridge for at least two hours.

Servings Provided: 1.5 dozen

Time Required: 50 minutes + chill time

Macro Counts - Each Serving:

- Calories: 153
- Carbs: 19 g
- Fiber: -0- g
- Sugar: 12 g
- Chol: 31 mg
- Prot.: 4 g
- Sodium: 216 mg
- Fat Content: 7 g (Saturated: 4 g)
  D.E.:
- Starch: 1
- Fat: 1 ½

Ingredients Needed:

- Unchilled butter - softened (1/3 cup)
- Lemon juice - divided (4 tbsp.)
- A.P. flour (1.25 cups)
- Sugar - divided (1 cup)
- Salt (.5 tsp.)
- Cream cheese - reduced-fat (8 oz. pkg.)
- Cream cheese - fat-free (8 oz. pkg.)
- Egg (1 large)
- Grated lemon zest (2 tsp.)
- Raspberries (18 fresh - halved)
- Needed: 9-inch square pan

Preparation Technique:

1. Line the baking pan with foil and coat with a spritz of cooking oil spray. Place the pan to the side for now.

2. Mix the butter with ¼ cup sugar until smooth (2 min.). Stir in two tablespoons lemon juice. Mix in the flour and salt. Press into the covered pan.

3. Bake at 350° Fahrenheit or 177 ° Celsius until the edges are nicely browned (14-16 min.).

4. Meanwhile, combine the cream cheeses and remaining sugar until smooth. Add in the whisked egg, beating using the low-speed setting just until combined. Mix in lemon zest and the rest of the lemon juice. Empty it over the crust.

5. Bake until filling is set (14-18 min.).

6. Let it cool on a wire rack for one hour. Pop it into the fridge for about two hours. Using foil, lift bars out of the pan. Gently peel off the layer of foil and cut them into squares, then triangles. Top it off using the raspberries.

Chapter 12

Candy & Other Tasty Favorites

Servings Provided: 15

Time Required: 10 minutes

Macro Counts - Each Serving:

- Calories: 70
- Carbs: 9 g
- Sugar: 6 g
- Fiber: 1 g
- Chol: 1 mg
- Prot.: 3 g
- Sodium: 46 mg
- Fat Content: 3 g (Saturated: 1 g)
  D.E.:
- Starch: ½
- Fat: ½

Ingredients Needed:

- Chunky peanut butter (.33 cup)
- Honey (.25 cup)
- Vanilla extract (.5 tsp.)
- Quick-cooking oats (.33 cup)
- Nonfat dry milk powder (.33 cup)
- Graham cracker crumbs (2 tbsp.)

Preparation Technique:

1. Cream the peanut butter with the honey and vanilla. Mix in the milk powder, oats, and cracker crumbs.
2. Shape the mixture into one-inch balls. Cover and pop them into the fridge until it's time to serve.

Servings Provided: 1.5 dozen

Time Required: 1 hour 40 minutes + cool time

Macro Counts - Each Serving:

- Calories: 32
- Carbs: 8 g
- Sugar: 7 g
- Chol: -0- mg
- Sodium: 23 mg
- Fat Content: -0- g
  D.E.:
- Starch: ½

Ingredients Needed:

- Egg whites, room temperature (2 large)
- Salt (.125 tsp.)
- Sugar (.5 cup)
- Cream of tartar (.125 tsp.)
- Peppermint candy canes (2 crushed)

Preparation Technique:

1. Beat the egg whites until foamy. Sprinkle in the cream of tartar and salt, mixing until you reach the soft peak stage.
2. Slowly mix in the sugar to reach stiff peaks (7 min.). Drop the mixture by teaspoonfuls onto paper or foil-lined baking sheets. Decorate them using the crushed candy.
3. Bake at 225° Fahrenheit or 107° Celsius for 1.5 hours.
4. Extinguish the oven's heat and leave the cookies with the door slightly open until cooled (1 hr.).
5. Keep them in a closed container.

Servings Provided: 8 (1.25 cups sauce)

Time Required: 15 minutes + chill time

Macro Counts - Each Serving:

- Calories: 176
- Carbs: 33 g
- Fiber: 2 g
- Sugar: 30 g
- Chol: 1 mg
- Fat Content: -0- g (Saturated: -0- g)
- Sodium: 37 mg
- Protein: 3 g

Ingredients Needed:

- Unflavored gelatin (1 envelope)
- Water - cold (.75 cup)
- Sugar (.66 cup)
- Vanilla extract (1 tsp.)
- Sour cream - fat-free (1 cup)
- Whipped topping - fat-free (2 cups)
- The Sauce:
- Frozen sweetened raspberries or sliced strawberries - thawed (10 oz. pkg.)
- Cornstarch (1 tbsp.)
- Sugar (1 tbsp.)

Preparation Technique:

1. Prepare a saucepan, and sprinkle the gelatin into cold water. Wait for one minute. Add sugar and warm it while stirring using the low-temperature setting until the gelatin and sugar are liquified.
2. Transfer the mixture into a bowl. Whisk in sour cream and vanilla and refrigerate it for ten minutes.

3. Mix in the whipped topping. Empty it into a four-cup mold coated with cooking spray. Refrigerate, covered, until firm, about four hours.

4. Prepare the sauce by draining the berries, reserving the syrup. Pour in enough water to the syrup to measure ¾ cup.

5. Use a small saucepan to mix the cornstarch with the sugar and syrup mixture until smooth. Once boiling, simmer and stir until thickened (2 min.). Cool slightly. Stir in drained berries and refrigerate until serving.

6. To serve, unmold dessert onto a serving plate. Serve with sauce.

Keto-Friendly Fat Bombs

Servings Provided: 12

Time Required: 25 minutes

Macro Counts - Each Serving:

- Calories: 194
- Carbs: 3.5 g
- Fiber: 1.5 g
- Sugar: 0.3 g
- Chol: 3.2 mg
- Protein: 3.8 g
- Sodium: 1.1 mg
- Fat Content: 16.8 g (Saturated: 10 g)
- Net Carbs: 2 g

Ingredients Needed:

- Unsweetened Cacao/cocoa powder (.25 cup/21 g)
- Natural chunky peanut butter (5 tbsp.)
- Shelled hemp seeds (6 tbsp.)
- Heavy cream (2 tbsp.)
- Unchilled-unrefined coconut oil (.5 cup/100 g)
- Vanilla extract (1 tsp.)
- Stevia (2 tbsp.)

Preparation Technique:

1. Mix the cocoa powder with the hemp seeds and peanut butter in a large mixing container.
2. Mix in the oil until it is pasty. Fold in the vanilla, stevia, and cream - sitting until it's a paste once again.
3. Roll the mixture into balls. (If the paste is too thin to roll, pop it in the fridge for ½ hour before proceeding.) Roll them in shredded coconut.

4. Arrange the balls on a layer of parchment baking paper on a cookie tin.

5. Freeze for ten minutes or leave them in the fridge for a minimum of 30 minutes before serving.

Servings Provided: 12

Time Required: 10 minutes prep - 1 .5 hours wait time

Macro Counts - Per Serving:

- ½ bomb = 1 serving:
- Calories: 247
- Carbohydrates: 247 g
- Sugar: 0.5 g
- Fiber: 1.2 g
- Prot.: 3.6 g
- Chol: -0- mg
- Sodium: 101.7 mg
- Fat Content: 24.4 g (Saturated: 15.3 g)

Ingredients Needed:

- The Bombs:
- Coconut oil (.5 cup/100 g)
- Peanut butter - no added salt or sugar (.75 cup/185 g)
- Sea salt (.25 tsp.)
- Vanilla extract (1 tsp.)
- Liquid stevia (3-4 drops)
- The Ganache:
- Cocoa powder (1 tbsp.)
- Coconut oil (6 tbsp.)
- Liquid stevia/favorite sweetener (1-2 drops)
- Also Needed: Six-count muffin tray

Preparation Technique:

1. Use a small bowl to melt the coconut oil and combine it with the peanut butter, stevia sweetener, vanilla extract, and salt. Heat in the microwave briefly and whisk until creamy.

2. Prepare the muffin tray with paper cups. Spoon the peanut butter mixture into each cup (3 tbsp. each).
3. Pop them in the fridge for at least one hour to overnight until firm.
4. Meanwhile, whisk the ganache ingredients until smooth.
5. Spoon about one tablespoon of the ganache over each fat bomb.
6. Chill for at least 30 minutes in the fridge before serving.
7. Enjoy them for up to one week stored in the fridge.

Chapter 13

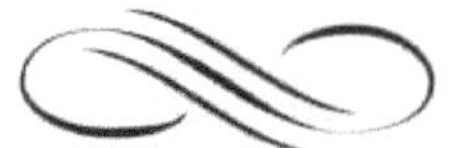

Beverages

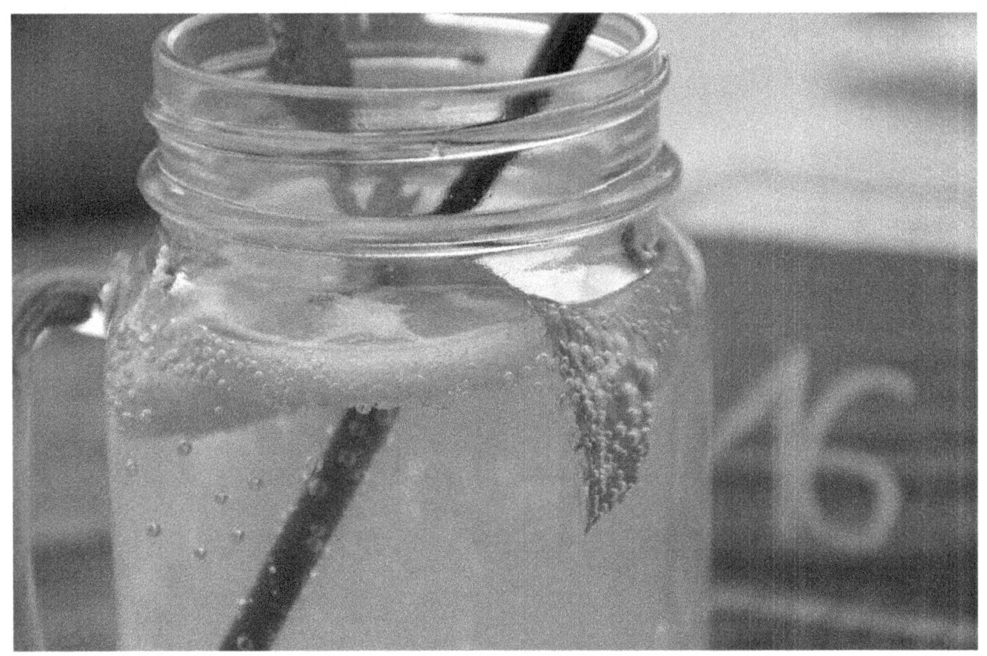

Servings Provided: 6

Time Required: 20 minutes

Macro Counts - Each Serving:

- ¾ cup portion:
- Calories: 98
- Fiber: 0.3 g
- Carbs: 26.8 g
- Sugar: 24.3 g
- Prot.: 0.5 g
- Sodium: 5.5 mg

- Fat Content: 0.2 g

  D.E.:

- Other Carbohydrate: 1 ½

Ingredients Needed:

- Fresh lemon juice (1.25 cups/+ more for garnishing/from about 8 lemons)
- Honey/agave syrup (.5 cup)
- Packed fresh basil leaves (1 cup + more to garnish)
- Water (3 cups - cold)
- Ice cubes (1 cup)

Preparation Technique:

- Load the blender with the basil, honey, and lemon juice, mixing until it's creamy smooth. Pour it into a large jar or pitcher using a sieve to strain.
- Pour in the water and pop it into the fridge until time to serve.
- Enjoy it over ice and a lemon slice with a couple of basil leaves.

Servings Provided: 6

Time Required: 5 minutes

Macro Counts - Each Serving:

- ☐ Calories: 23
- ☐ Sugar: 2 g
- ☐ Sodium: 10 mg
- ☐ Net Carbs: 6 g

Ingredients Needed:

- ☐ Lemon (1)
- ☐ Lime (1)
- ☐ Orange (1)
- ☐ Pink grapefruit (1)
- ☐ Water (6 cups)

Preparation Technique:

1. Slice each piece of fruit into halves.
2. Juice all of the fruit into a measuring cup and trash the rinds.
3. Pour the juice through a strainer and into a pitcher that will hold at least 8 cups of liquid.
4. Add the water and stir well to serve.

Servings Provided: 6

Time Required: 5 minutes

Macro Counts - Each Serving:

- ☐ Calories: 23
- ☐ Carbs: 6 g
- ☐ Sugar: 5.5 g
- ☐ Sodium: 38.7 mg
  D.E.: Fruit: ½

Ingredients Needed:

- ☐ Ice cubes (1 cup)
- ☐ Low-calorie grape/cranberry or pomegranate juice (3 cups)
- ☐ Sparkling water (3 cups)
- ☐ Optional: Halved fresh cranberries, grapes, or raspberries (.75 cup)

Preparation Technique:

1. Half fill six tall glasses with ice cubes.
2. Portion the grape juice evenly between the glasses.
3. Pour sparkling water into the glasses, and gently stir.
4. Decorate with a few floating grapes in the drinks.

Servings Provided: 5

Time Required: 20 minutes

Macro Counts - Each Serving:

- ☐ Calories: 3
- ☐ Protein: 0.5 g
- ☐ Sodium: 2.9mg
- ☐ Saturated: -0- g
- ☐ Free exchanges

Ingredients Needed:

- ☐ Water (6 cups)
- ☐ Sugar substitute (1 tbsp.)
- ☐ Lemon peel (8 strips)
- ☐ Fresh ginger (2-inch piece)
- ☐ Green tea bags (3)
- ☐ Lemon (5 slices)

Preparation Technique:

1. Slice the lemon strips (2.5 x 1-inches). Peel and thinly slice the ginger.
2. Prepare a saucepan of water and toss in the strips of lemon and ginger. Lower the temperature setting, and simmer for ten minutes. Discard the ginger and lemon.
3. Toss the tea bags in a teapot and promptly add to the simmering lemon-infused water. Place a lid on the pot and steep for one to three minutes. Remove the tea bags, squeezing gently.
4. Serve right away in heatproof glass mugs or cups. Sweeten as desired using your favorite sugar substitute and serve with lemon slices.
5. Tip: Remove lemon peel with a vegetable peeler. If necessary, use a sharp knife to scrape off any white pith that remains on the peel, as this can cause bitterness.

Servings Provided: 4

Time Required: 5 minutes

Macro Counts - Each Serving:

- Calories: 47
- Fiber: 0.5 g
- Sugar: 11.7 g
- Carbs: 0.2 g
- Chol: -0- mg
- Sodium: 24.3 mg
- Fat Content: -0- g
- D.E.: Other Carbohydrate: 1

Ingredients Needed:

- Ice - divided (2 cups)
- Diet cranberry juice drink - divided (1.33 cups)
- Peach nectar, divided (1.33 cups)
- Mint (4 sprigs)
- Quartered orange (4 slices)

Preparation Technique:

1. Put ½ cup of ice into each of the glasses.
2. Add 1/3 cup portions of cranberry juice and peach nectar to each glass.
3. Top them off with mint springs and orange slices.

Servings Provided: 6 cups

Time Required: 5 minutes

Macro Counts - Each Serving:

- Calories: 16
- Fiber: 1 g
- Carbs: 4 g
- Sugar: 3 g
- Sodium: 30 mg
- Fat Content: -0- g
- Prot.: 0.3 g
- Net Carbs: 3 g

Ingredients Needed:

- Fresh strawberries (2 cups)
- Water (4 cups)
- Kosher salt (1 pinch)
- Optional: Honey or another sweetener (1 tbsp.)

Preparation Technique:

1. Place the strawberries, water, salt, and sweetener into a blender.
2. Purée until smooth.
3. Serve in chilled glasses.

Diabetic-Friendly Cocktails & Mocktails

Servings Provided: 6

Time Required: 15 minutes

Macro Counts - Each Serving:

- ☐ Calories: 152
- ☐ Fiber: 0.3 g
- ☐ Carbs: 12.6g
- ☐ Sugar: 9.8 g
- ☐ Prot.: 0.4 g
- ☐ Sodium: 1.9 mg
- ☐ Fat Content: 0.1 g (Saturated: -0- g)
  D.E.:
- ☐ Alcohol Equivalent: 1
- ☐ Fruit: ½

Ingredients Needed:

- ☐ Grated blood orange zest (1 tbsp.)
- ☐ Optional: Kosher salt (1 tbsp.)
- ☐ Blood orange juice (1 cup)
- ☐ White tequila (1 cup)
- ☐ Lime juice (.5 cup + 1 lime wedge)
- ☐ Triple Sec (.25 cup)
- ☐ Simple syrup (2 tbsp.)
- ☐ Ice cubes (1 cup)
- ☐ To Garnish:
- ☐ Blood orange slices (6 slices)
- ☐ Lime slices (12 slices)

Preparation Technique:

1. Chill the tequila and orange juice.

2. Sprinkle orange zest on a small plate and combine with salt (if using).

3. Mix the tequila with the lime juice, simple syrup, orange juice, and Triple Sec in a pitcher.

4. Rub the rims of six glasses with the lime wedge and dip in the zest (or zest-salt mixture).

5. Fill each of the glasses with ice and pour in about ½ cup of the margarita mixture into each. Top it off with lime or orange slices as desired.

Servings Provided: 8

Time Required: 25 minutes

Macro Counts - Each Serving:

- Calories: 184
- Carbs: 30 g
- Sugar: 29 g
- Sodium: 0.3 mg
- Fat Content: -0- g
- **D.E.:**
- Fruit: 2

Ingredients Needed:

- Apple cider/apple juice (8 cups)
- Whole allspice berries (4)
- Whole cloves (4)
- Whole cardamom seeds (4)
- Cinnamon (4 sticks)
- Calvados - brandy (1 cup)

Preparation Technique:

1. Combine the cider or juice with the cloves, cardamom, allspice, and cinnamon sticks in a large saucepan.
2. Simmer for 20 minutes and strain out the spices
3. Stir in the Calvados or brandy.
4. Serve piping-hot in heavy mugs.

Servings Provided: 6

Time Required: 15 minutes

Macro Counts - Each Serving:

- 2/3 Cup Cocoa & 1.5 Tablespoons Topper:
- Calories: 203
- Carbs: 23.5 g
- Fiber: 2.1 g
- Sugar: 19.8 g
- Chol: 3.3 mg
- Prot.: 7.2 g
- Sodium: 69.8 mg
- Fat Content: 6.3 g (Saturated: 3.7 g)
  D.E.:
- Starch: ½
- Fat: 2
- Other Carbohydrate: ½
- Milk: ½

Ingredients Needed:

- Bittersweet chocolate pieces (.5 cup)
- Unsweetened cocoa powder (.25 cup)
- Fat-free milk (4 cups)
- Honey (2 tbsp.)
- Bourbon (.5 cup/4 oz.)
- Ground cinnamon (1 pinch)

Preparation Technique:

1. Melt the chocolate pieces and cocoa powder in a saucepan.
2. Whisk in 3.5 cups of the milk and the honey.
3. Simmer using the medium-temperature setting, just until boiling and chocolate pieces are melted, whisking constantly. Stir in the bourbon.

4. For a frothy topper, pour the rest of the milk (.5 cup) into a medium bowl. Microwave 20-30 seconds or until warm. Beat with a whisk until frothy.

5. Serve the cocoa with a frothy topper and a sprinkle of cinnamon or more cocoa powder.

Servings Provided: 4

Time Required: 10 minutes

Macro Counts - Each Serving:

- Calories: 124
- Carbs: 33.5 g
- Sugar: 26.5 g
- Prot.: 0.8 g
- Fat Content: 0.2 g (Saturated: -0- g)
- Sodium: 6.1 mg
- D.E.:Starch: Other Carbohydrate: 1 ½

Ingredients Needed:

- Fresh lime juice (.75 cup/from 6 limes)
- Simple syrup (.75 cup **)
- Packed fresh mint leaves (.5 cup)
- Lime zest (2 strips - 2-inch)
- Ice cubes (4 cups)
- Sparkling water (2 cups)
- To Garnish: Lime slices (4 slices @ ¼-inch thickness) & mint sprigs (4)

Preparation Technique:

1. Make your simple syrup: **Pour one cup of sugar into a medium saucepan, frequently stirring until it's liquified. Cool the mixture for ½ hour and refrigerate until cold (1 hr.). Simple syrup can be stored in the fridge, covered, for up to six months.
2. Combine the lime juice, simple syrup, mint leaves, and lime zest in a pitcher. Lightly crush the mint and zest.
3. Add ice cubes and sparkling water, thoroughly stirring to serve.
4. Portion the drink into four glasses. Garnish with lime slices and mint sprigs, as desired.

Servings Provided: 1 serving or 1.5 cups

Time Required: 1 hour 40 minutes

Macro Counts - Each Serving:

- ☐ 5 fl oz. portion:
- ☐ Calories: 126
- ☐ Carbs: 11.1 g
- ☐ Sugar: 8.8 g
- ☐ Fiber: 0.1 g
- ☐ Chol: -0- mg
- ☐ Prot.: 0.4 g
- ☐ Sodium: 0.5 mg
- ☐ Fat Content: -0- g
  D.E.:
- ☐ Other Carbohydrates: ½
- ☐ Fat: 2

Ingredients Needed:

- ☐ The Simple Syrup:
- ☐ Sugar (1 cup)
- ☐ Water (1 cup)
- ☐ The Cocktail:
- ☐ Fresh lemon juice (.5 oz.)
- ☐ Chilled sparkling wine - ex. - Prosecco (4 oz.)
- ☐ Simple Syrup ↑ (.5 oz.)
- ☐ To Garnish: 1 Lemon twist

Preparation Technique:

- ☐ Make the simple syrup by bringing the water and sugar to a boil in a saucepan, frequently stirring to liquefy the sugar. Cool it for ½ hour and refrigerate until cold (1 hr.).

□ To prepare an individual cocktail: Combine ½ oz. of the simple syrup and lemon juice in a champagne flute.

□ Top it off using sparkling wine and garnish with a lemon twist.

Conclusion

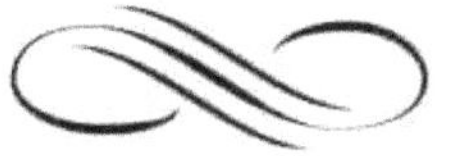

I hope you have thoroughly enjoyed each of the recipes provided in your new copy of the Diabetic Desserts for Beginners. I hope it was informative and provided you with all of the tools you need to achieve your goals, whatever they may be.

The next step is to head to the market and prepare one of the delicious options for dessert tonight!

The experts state you don't need to eliminate all sugar. However, many will eventually consume more sugar than is healthy. You need to learn moderation, especially if you have diabetes. Thus, you'll find this cookbook will be your best friend, so you can enjoy your favorite dessert once in a while.

It takes time for your taste buds to adjust once you begin to reduce your intake of sugar. Thus, your cravings should also diminish.

When you want to enjoy dessert, eliminate that portion of pasta, rice, or bread. It is all in working the carbohydrates to your advantage, instead of making it difficult to pack the meal with both options.

Consider adding more healthy fat as you enjoy dessert. Fat will slow down the digestive process, which means your blood sugar levels won't spike quickly. However, you shouldn't reach for the donuts. Envision healthier fats, such as ricotta cheese, yogurt, peanut butter, or nuts.

Save your sweets for mealtime, not a mid-afternoon snack. When eaten solo, sweets will cause your blood sugar to spike. However, if you eat them with other healthy foods as part of your meal, your blood sugar will not rise as rapidly.

Enjoy every morsel of your special dessert dish. Eat slowly and indulge in its flavor. Not only will the food be more enjoyable, but you are also less likely to overeat.

I sincerely hope you have found the information useful. Finally, if you found this book helpful in any way, a review on Amazon is always appreciated!

DIABETICS DIET COOKBOOKS AFTER 50

COMPLETE GUIDE ON HOW TO LOSE WEIGHT WITH INGREDIENT AND SIMPLE RECIPE WITH LOW CARBOHYDRATE

INTRODUCTION ON HEALTHY EATING

Eating well is fundamental to good health and well-being. Healthy eating helps us to maintain a healthy weight. It reduces our risk of diabetes, high blood pressure, high cholesterol, and the risk of developing cardiovascular disease and some cancers.

WHY IS EATING WELL IMPORTANT?

Healthy eating has many other benefits. When we eat well, we sleep better, have more energy, and better concentration – and this all adds up to healthier, happier lives! Healthy eating should be an enjoyable social experience. When children and young people eat and drink well, they get all the essential nutrients they need to develop and develop a good relationship with food and other social skills.

What is healthy eating?

Healthy eating isn't about cutting out foods – it's about eating a wide variety of foods in the right amounts to give your body what it needs. There are no available foods you must eat or menus you need to follow to eat healthily. You just need to make sure you get the right balance of different foods. Healthy eating for children and young people should always include a range of exciting and tasty food that can make up a healthy, varied, and balanced diet, rather than denying them certain foods and drinks. Although all foods can be included in a healthy diet, this will not be true for special/medical diets.

What are the benefits of eating healthy?

A healthful diet includes various fruits and vegetables of many colors, whole grains and starches, good fats, and lean proteins. Eating healthfully also means avoiding foods with high amounts of added salt and sugar.

We look at the top 10 benefits of a healthful diet, as well as the evidence behind them.

1. Weight loss

Losing weight can help to reduce the risk of chronic conditions. If a person is overweight or obese, they have a higher risk of developing several conditions, including:

- Heart Disease
- Non-Insulin-Dependent Diabetes Mellitus
- Poor Bone Density
- Some Cancers

Whole vegetables and fruits are lower in calories than most processed foods. A person looking to lose weight should reduce their calorie intake to no more than what they require each day.

Maintaining a healthful diet free from processed foods can help a person stay within their daily limit without counting calories. Fiber is one element of a healthful diet that is particularly important for managing weight. Plant-based foods contain plenty of dietary FiberFiber, regulating hunger by making people feel fuller for longer.

In 2018, researchers found that a diet rich in FiberFiber and lean proteins resulted in weight loss without the need for counting calories.

2. Reduced cancer risk

An unhealthful diet can lead to obesity, which may increase a person's risk of developing cancer. Weighing within a healthful range may reduce this risk.

In 2014, the American Society of Clinical Oncology reported that obesity contributed to a worse outlook for people with cancer.

However, diets rich in fruits and vegetables may help to protect against cancer.

In a separate study from 2014, researchers found that a diet rich in fruits reduced the risk of cancers of the upper gastrointestinal tract. They also found that a diet rich in vegetables, fruits, and FiberFiber lowered the risk of colorectal cancer and that a diet rich in FiberFiber reduced the risk of liver cancer.

Many phytochemicals found in fruits, vegetables, nuts, and legumes act as antioxidants, which protect cells from damage that can cause cancer. Some of these antioxidants include beta-carotene, lycopene, and vitamins A, C, and E.

Trials in humans have been inconclusive, but results of laboratory and animal studies have linked certain antioxidants to a reduced incidence of free radical damage associated with cancer.

3. Diabetes management

Eating a healthful diet can help a person with diabetes to:

5. Lose Weight, If Re□uired

6. Manage Blood Glucose Levels
7. Keep Blood Pressure And Cholesterol Within Target Ranges Prevent Or Delay Complications Of Diabetes

It is essential for people with diabetes to limit their intake of foods with added sugar and salt. It is also best to avoid fried foods high in saturated and trans fats.

4. Heart health and stroke prevention

According to figures published in 2017, as many as 92.1 million people in the U.S. have at least one type of cardiovascular disease. These conditions primarily involve the heart or blood vessels.

According to the Heart and Stroke Foundation of Canada, up to 80 percent of premature heart disease and stroke cases can be prevented by making lifestyle changes, such as increasing levels of physical activity and eating healthfully.

There is some evidence that vitamin E may prevent blood clots, which can lead to heart attacks. The following foods contain high levels of vitamin E:

9. Almonds
10. Peanuts
11. Hazelnuts
12. Sunflower Seeds
13. Green Vegetables

The medical community has long recognized the link between trans fats and heart-related illnesses, such as coronary heart disease.

If a person eliminates trans fats from the diet, this will reduce their low-density lipoprotein cholesterol levels. This type of cholesterol causes plaque to collect within the arteries, increasing heart attack, and stroke risk.

Reducing blood pressure can also be essential for heart health, and limiting salt intake to 1,500 milligrams a day can help.

Salt is added to many processed and fast foods, and a person hoping to lower their blood pressure should avoid these.

5. The health of the next generation

Children learn most health-related behaviors from the adults around them, and parents who model healthful eating and exercise habits tend to pass these on.

Eating at home may also help. In 2018, researchers found that children who regularly had meals with their families ate more vegetables and fewer sugary foods than their peers who ate at home less freuently.

Also, children who participate in gardening and cooking at home may be more likely to make healthful dietary and lifestyle choices.

6. Strong bones and teeth

A diet with adeuate calcium and magnesium is necessary for strong bones and teeth. Keeping the bones healthy is vital in preventing osteoporosis and osteoarthritis later in life.

The following foods are rich in calcium:

- Low-Fat Dairy Products
- Broccoli
- Cauliflower
- Cabbage
- Canned Fish With Bones
- Tofu
- Legumes

Also, many bowls of cereal and plant-based milk are fortified with calcium.

Magnesium is abundant in many foods, and the best sources are leafy green vegetables, nuts, seeds, and whole grains.

7. Better mood

Emerging evidence suggests a close relationship between diet and mood.

In 2016, researchers found that a diet with a high glycemic load may increase depression and fatigue symptoms.

A diet with a high glycemic load includes many refined carbohydrates, such as those found in soft drinks, cakes, white bread, and biscuits. Vegetables, whole fruit, and whole grains have a lower glycemic load.

While a healthful diet may improve overall mood, people with depression need to seek medical care.

8. Improved memory

A healthful diet may help prevent dementia and cognitive decline.

A study from 2015 identified nutrients and foods that protect against these adverse effects. They found the following to be beneficial:

- Vitamin D, C, And E
- Omega-3 Fatty Acids
- Flavonoids And Polyphenols
- Fish

Among other diets, the Mediterranean diet incorporates many of these nutrients.

9. Improved gut health

The colon is full of naturally occurring bacteria, which play essential roles in metabolism and digestion.

Certain strains of bacteria also produce vitamins K and B, which benefit the colon. These strains also help to fight harmful bacteria and viruses.

A diet low in FiberFiber and high in sugar and fat alters the gut microbiome, increasing inflammation in the area.

However, a diet rich in vegetables, fruits, legumes, and whole grains provides a combination of prebiotics and probiotics that help good bacteria to thrive in the colon.

Fermented foods, such as Yogurt, kimchi, sauerkraut, miso, and kefir, are rich in probiotics. Fiber is an easily accessible prebiotic, and it is abundant in legumes, grains, fruits, and vegetables.

Fiber also promotes regular bowel movements, which can help to prevent bowel cancer and diverticulitis.

10. Getting a good night's sleep

A variety of factors, including sleep apnea, can disrupt sleep patterns.

Sleep apnea occurs when the airways are repeatedly blocked during sleep. Risk factors include obesity, drinking alcohol, and eating an unhealthy diet.

Reducing alcohol and caffeine consumption can help to ensure restful sleep, whether or not a person has sleep apnea.

Quick tips for a healthful diet

There are plenty of small, positive ways to improve the diet, including:

10. Swapping Soft Drinks For Water And Herbal Tea
11. Eating No Meat For At Least One Day A Week
12. Ensuring That Produce Makes Up About 50 Percent Of Each Meal

13. Swapping Cow's Milk For Plant-Based Milk

14. Eating Whole Fruits Instead Of Drinking Juices, Which Contain Less Fiberfiber And Often Include Added Sugar

15. Avoiding Processed Meats, Which Are High In Salt And May Increase The Risk Of Colon Cancer

16. Eating More Lean Protein, Which Can Be Found In Eggs, Tofu, Fish, And Nuts

A person may also benefit from taking a cooking class and learning how to incorporate more vegetables into meals. A doctor or dietitian can also provide tips on eating a more healthful diet.

A GUIDE TO HEALTHY LOW CARB EATING WITH DIABETES

Diabetes is a chronic disease that affects many people across the globe. Currently, more than 400 million people have diabetes worldwide.

Although diabetes is a complicated disease, maintaining adequate blood sugar levels can significantly reduce the risk of complications.

One of the ways to achieve better blood sugar levels is to follow a low carb diet. This article provides a detailed overview of deficient carb diets for managing diabetes. With diabetes, the body can't effectively process carbohydrates.

Usually, when you eat carbs, they're broken down into small glucose units, which end up as blood sugar. When blood sugar levels go up, the pancreas responds by producing the hormone insulin. This hormone allows blood sugar to enter cells.

What IS DIABETES, AND WHAT ROLE DOES FOOD PLAY?

With diabetes, the body can't effectively process carbohydrates. Usually, when you eat carbs, they're broken down into small glucose units, which end up as blood sugar.

When blood sugar levels go up, the pancreas responds by producing the hormone insulin. This hormone allows blood sugar to enter cells. In people without diabetes, blood sugar levels remain within a narrow range throughout the day. For those who have diabetes, however, this system doesn't work in the same way. This is a big problem because having both too high and too low blood sugar levels can cause severe harm.

There are several types of diabetes, but the two most common ones are type 1 and type 2 diabetes. Both of these conditions can occur at any age.

In type 1 diabetes, an autoimmune process destroys the insulin-producing beta cells in the pancreas. People with diabetes take insulin several times a day to ensure that glucose gets into the cells and stays healthy in the bloodstream.

In type 2 diabetes, the beta cells at first produce enough insulin, but the body's cells are resistant to its action, so blood sugar remains high. To compensate, the pancreas produces more insulin, attempting to bring blood sugar down.

Over time, the beta cells lose their ability to produce enough insulin. Of the three macronutrients — protein, carbs, and fat — carbs significantly impact blood sugar management. This is because the body breaks them down into glucose. Therefore, people with diabetes may need to take large doses of insulin, medication, or both when they eat many carbohydrates.

Can Deficient Carb Diets Help Manage Diabetes?

Many studies support low carb diets for the treatment of diabetes. In fact, before discovering insulin in 1921, deficient carb diets were considered standard treatment for people with diabetes.

What's more, low carb diets seem to work well in the long term when people stick to them. In one study, people with type 2 diabetes ate a low carb diet for six months. Their diabetes remained well managed more than three years later if they stuck to the diet.

Similarly, when people with type 1 diabetes followed a carb-restricted diet, those who followed the diet saw a significant improvement in blood sugar levels over four years.

A LOW-CARB DIET AND MEALPLAN

Eating a low-carb diet means cutting down on the number of carbohydrates (carbs) you eat to less than 130g a day. But low-carb eating shouldn't be no-carb eating.

Some carbohydrate foods contain essential vitamins, minerals, and FiberFiber, which form an essential part of a healthy diet.

Here we'll explain what we mean by low-carb, the benefits of low-carb eating when you have diabetes, and share a low-carb meal plan to help you get started if this is the diet for you. We'll also explain how to get support to manage any potential risks, especially if you manage your diabetes with medications that put you at risk of hypos.

If you or someone you know is self-isolating, find out how to eat healthily while staying at home.

What's A Low-Carb Diet?

But how low is low-carb? There are different types of low-carb diets. Generally, low-carb eating reduces the total amount of carbs you consume in a day to less than 130g.

To put this into context, a medium-sized slice of bread is about 15 to 20g of carbs, which is about the same as a regular apple. On the other hand, a large jacket potato could have as much as 90g of carbs, as does one liter of orange juice.

A low-carb diet isn't for everyone. The most substantial evidence we have to show the benefits of low-carb diets is in adults with obesity and those with type 2 diabetes who need to lose weight. If you decide to follow a low-carb diet, it's essential to know all the potential benefits and manage any potential risks.

Low-Carb Meal Plan

There's no one-size-fits-all for choosing a meal plan. Before you begin any healthy eating program, please read our guide on choosing your meal plan to ensure you follow the plan that's right for you.

Our low-carb meal plan aims to help you maintain a healthy balance while reducing the number of carbs you eat. Varying amounts of carbohydrates are shown each day to help you choose which works best for you. It's nutritionally balanced, we've counted the calories for you, and it contains at least five portions of fruit and veg per day.

Low-Carb Diet

Monday's low-carb meal plan

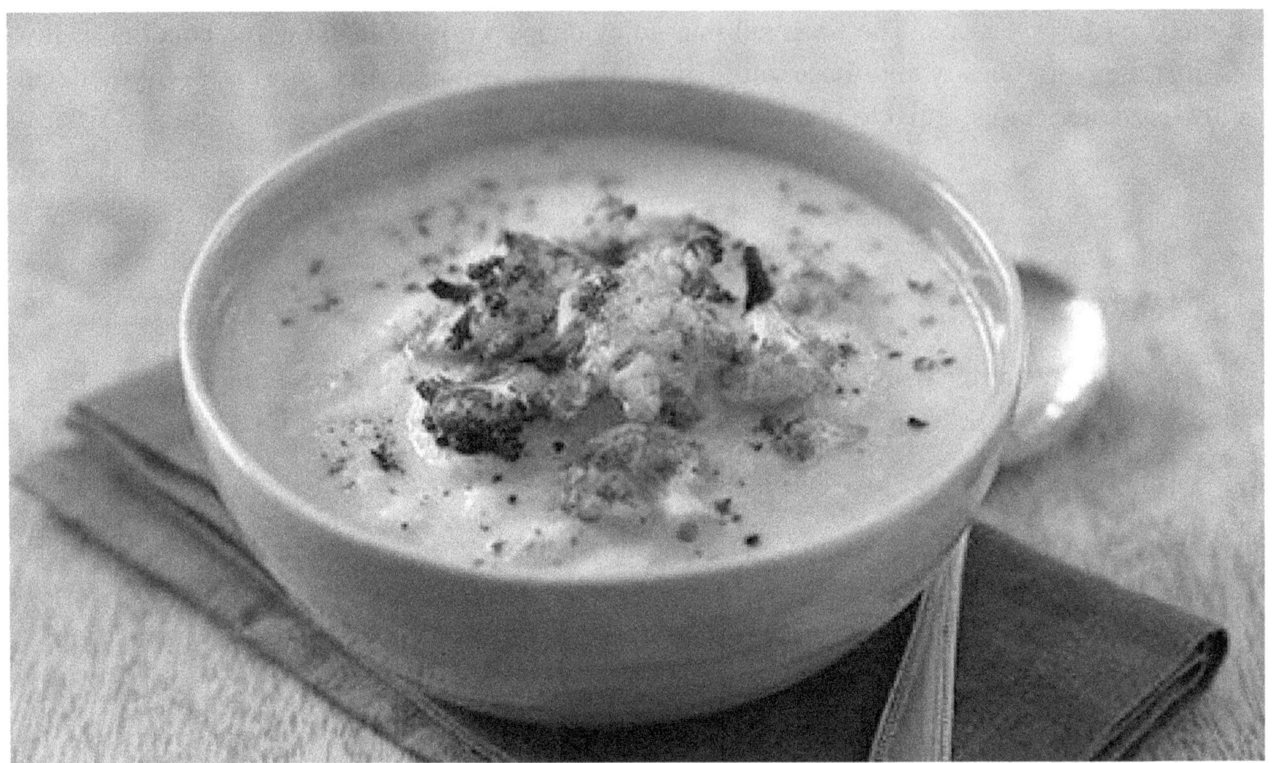

Breakfast: Wholemeal toast with scrambled eggs

Lunch: Cauliflower and leek soup

Dinner: Lower-fat Cauliflower and broccoli cheese with a medium grilled salmon fillet

Pudding: Greek Yogurt with raspberries

Choose from snacks, including fruit, nuts, and rye crackers with avocado.

Tuesday's low-carb meal plan

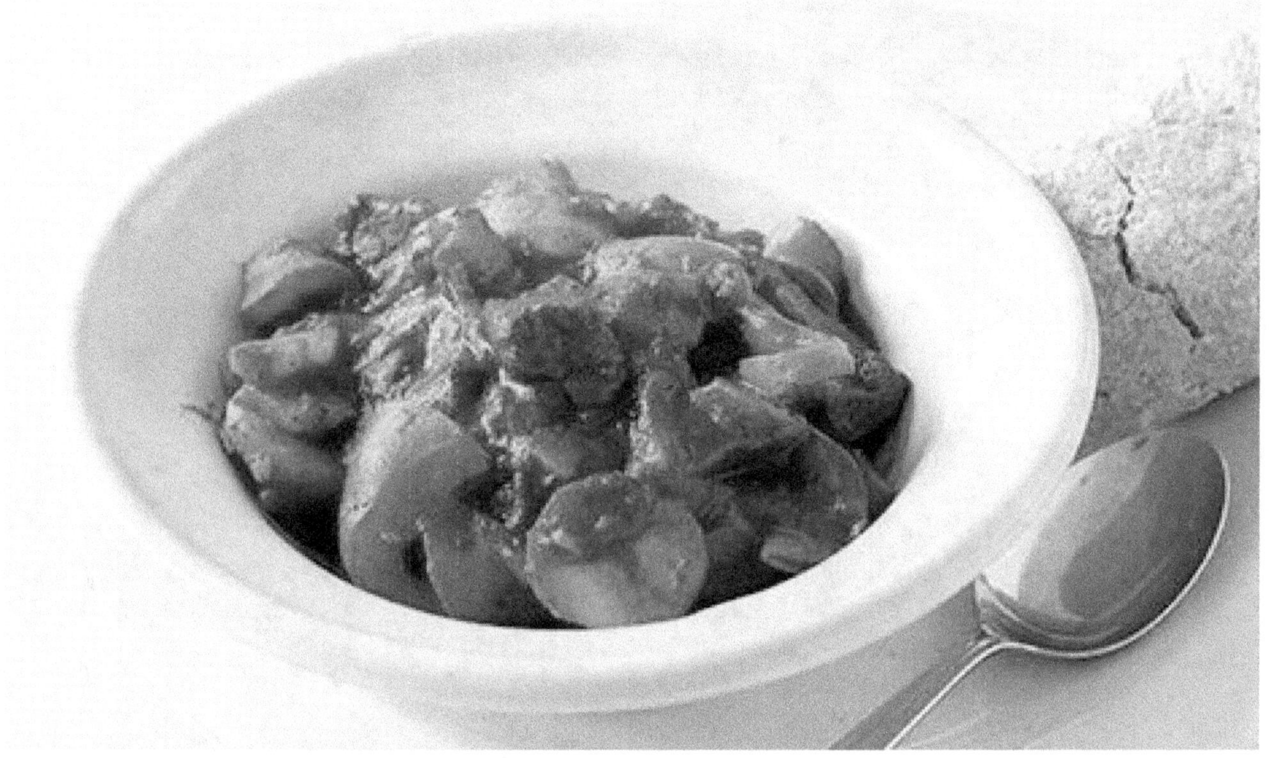

Breakfast: Greek Yogurt with raspberries and pumpkin seeds

Lunch: Chickpea and tuna salad and strawberries

Dinner: Beef goulash

Pudding: Rhubarb fool

Choose from snacks, including granary bread with peanut butter, avocado, Greek Yogurt, crudites, and nuts.

Wednesday's low-carb meal plan

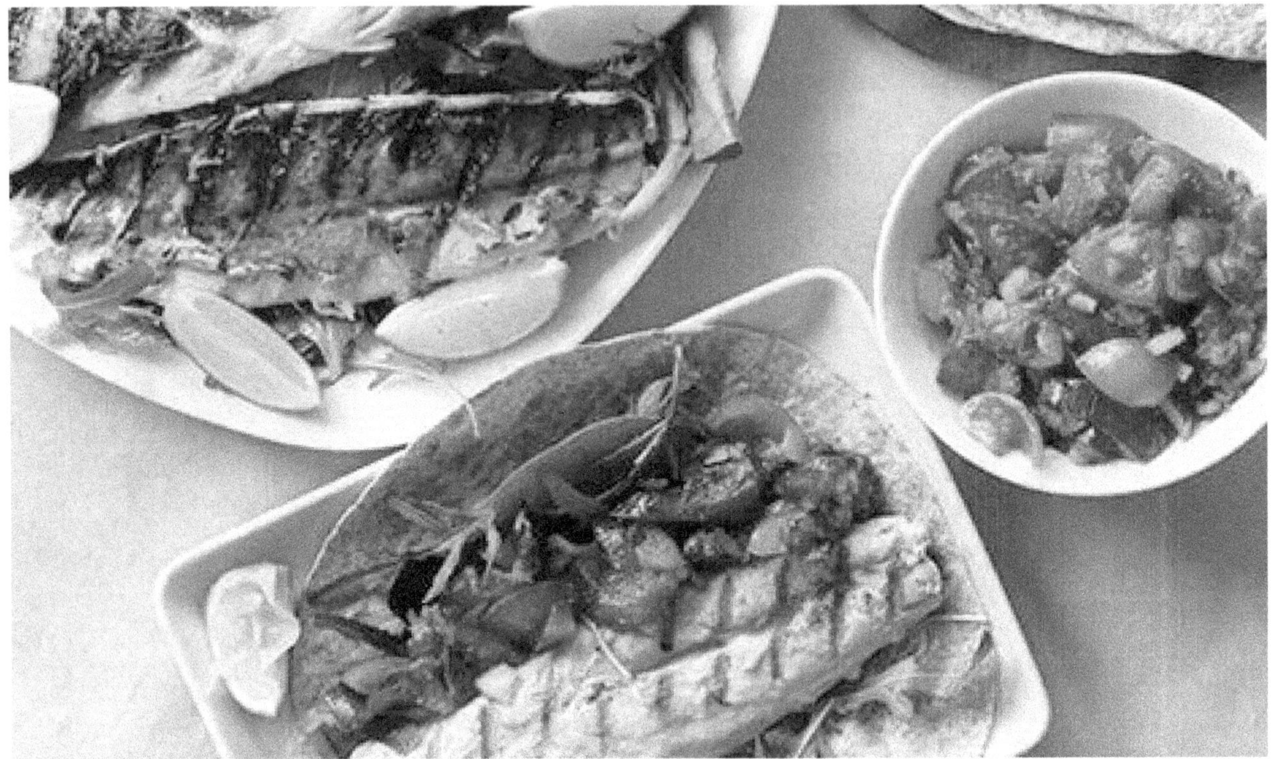

Breakfast: Porridge with almonds, blueberries, and pumpkin seeds

Lunch: Mackerel salsa wrap

Dinner: Chicken casserole with Broccoli

Pudding: Greek Yogurt with strawberries and blueberries

Choose from snacks, including nuts, wholemeal rice cakes with peanut butter, and crudites with guacamole.

Thursday's low-carb meal plan

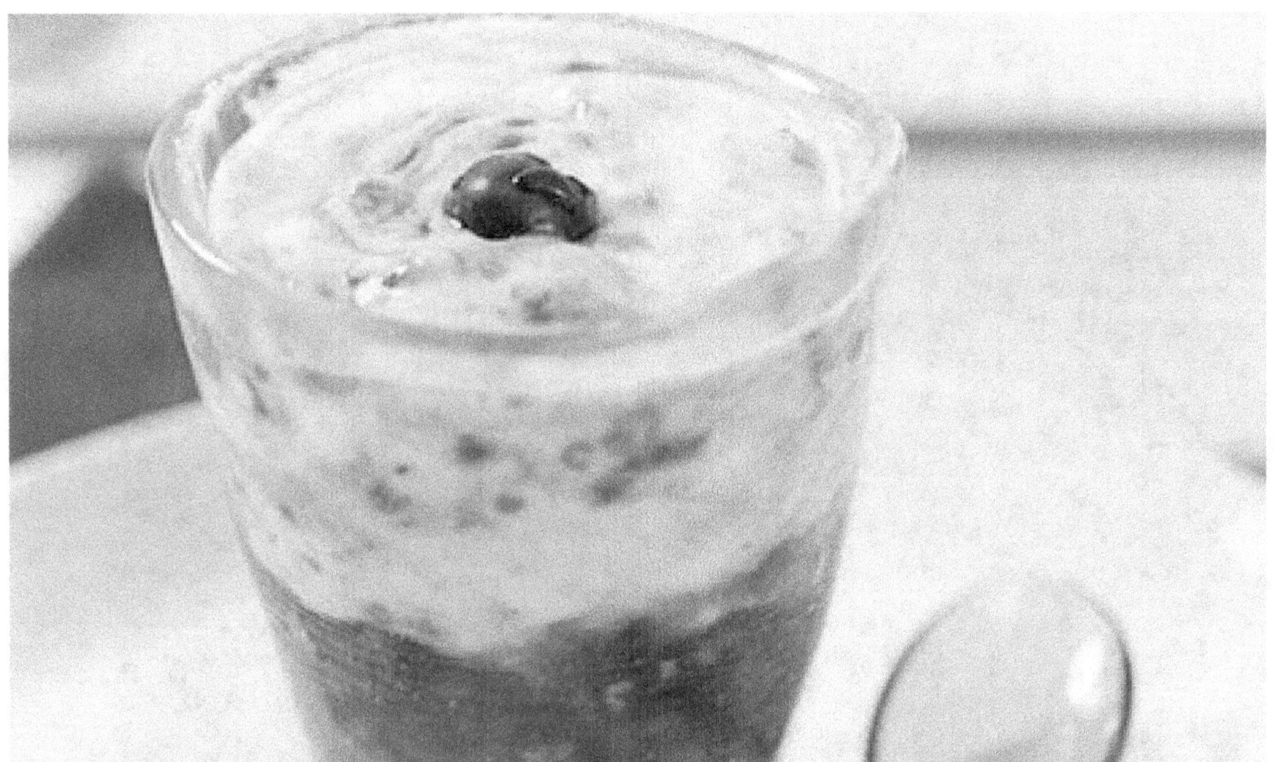

Breakfast: Mushroom omelet with mushrooms and grilled tomato

Lunch: Creamy chicken and mushroom soup and Greek Yogurt with raspberries

Dinner: Beefburger with a green salad

Pudding: Summer berry posset

Choose from snacks, including oatcakes with light cream cheese, nuts, and avocado.

Friday's low-carb meal plan

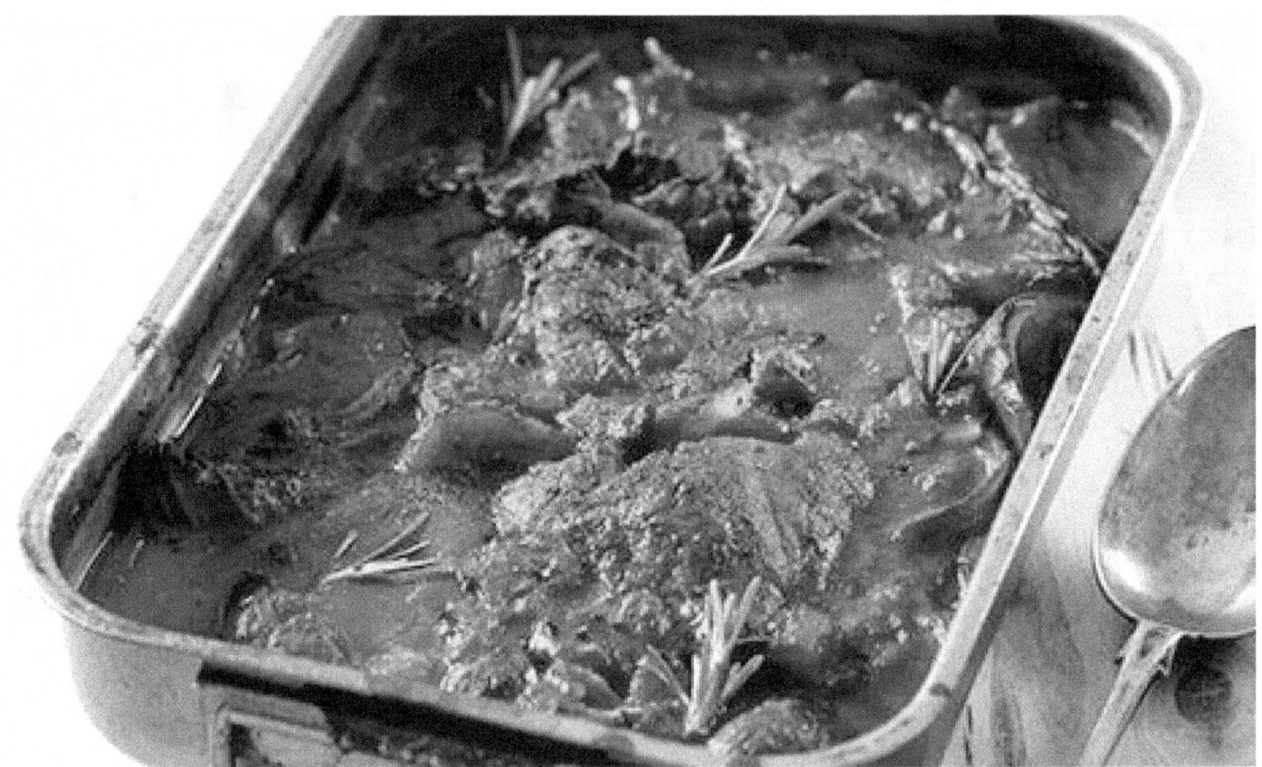

Breakfast: Scrambled egg on granary toast with mushrooms

Lunch: Beef and barley soup and Greek Yogurt

Dinner: Italian-style braised lamb steaks with brown rice and Broccoli

Pudding: Microwave mug: Chocolate, banana, and almond cup with half-fat creme fraiche

Choose from snacks, including nuts, cheese, and guacamole with crudites.

Saturday's low-carb meal plan

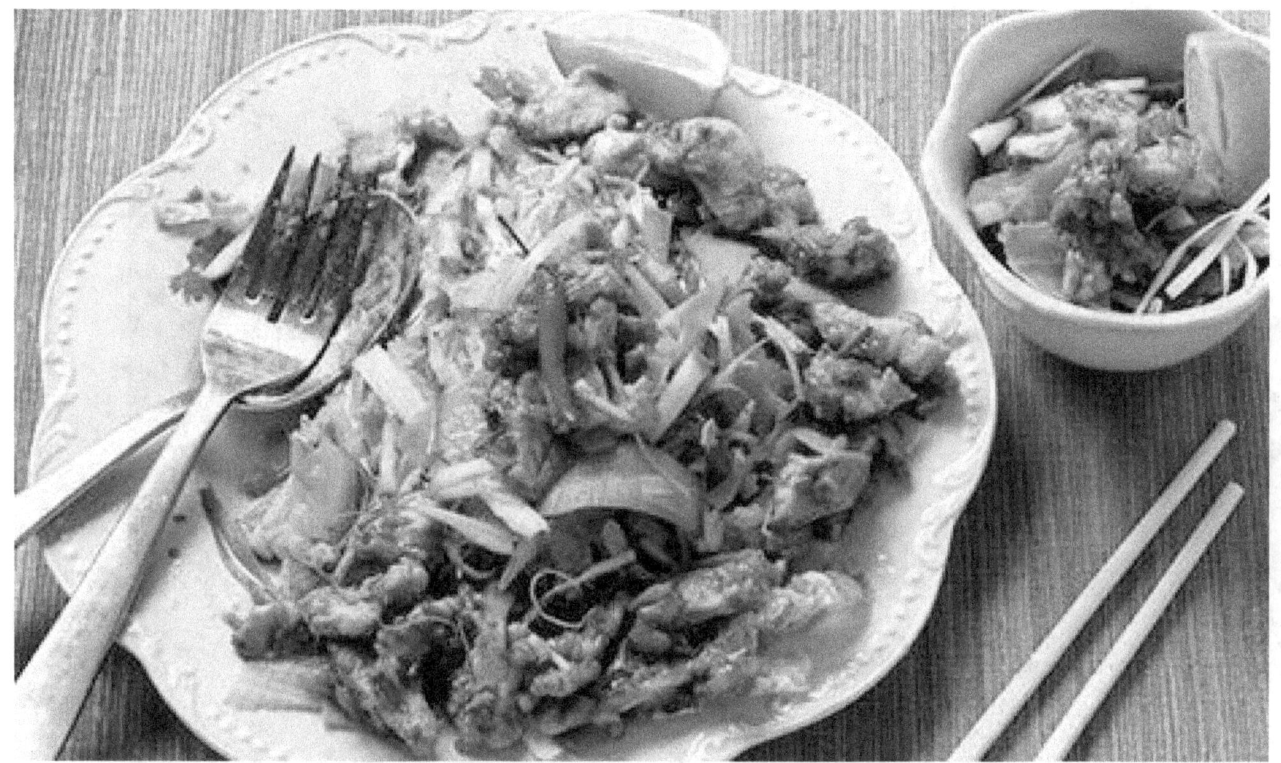

Breakfast: Wholemeal toast with grilled bacon and mushrooms

Lunch: Bang bang chicken salad

Dinner: Coq au vin with Broccoli

Pudding: Hot chocolate

Choose from snacks, including raspberry smoothie and nuts.

Sunday's low-carb meal plan

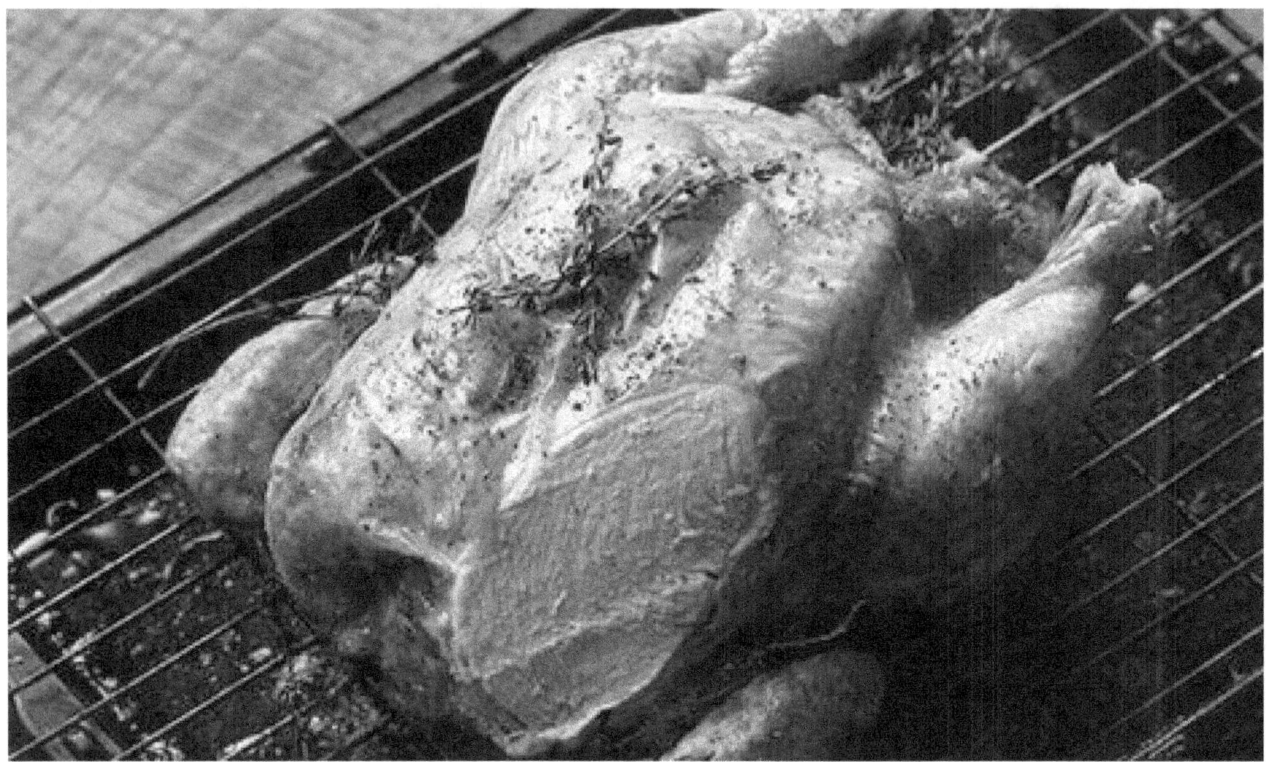

Breakfast: Scrambled egg with smoked salmon on granary toast

Lunch: Ham, leek, and Parmesan frittata with avocado, celery, cucumber, and lettuce

Dinner: Roast chicken, roast potatoes, green beans, and gravy

Pudding: Greek Yogurt with raspberries

Choose from snacks, including olives, nuts, dried fruit, and oatcakes with light cream cheese.

BENEFITS OF FOLLOWING A LOW-CARB DIET

One of the main benefits of following a low-carb diet is weight loss. For people with type 2 diabetes, this helps to reduce HbA1c and blood fats such as cholesterol. For people who don't have diabetes, losing weight can reduce your risk of developing type 2 diabetes, and a low-carb diet is one option to lose weight.

For people with type 1 diabetes

If you have type 1, it's essential to know that the best way to keep your blood sugar levels steady is to carb count rather than following a particular diet. And there is no substantial evidence that following a low-carb diet is safe or beneficial, which is why we don't recommend this diet for people with type 1 diabetes. But some people with type 1 have reported needing less insulin and losing weight from following a low-carb diet.

You must speak to your healthcare team for support to manage your insulin if you're considering a low-carb diet.

For people with type 2 diabetes

If you have type 2 diabetes, our research has shown that losing around 15kg within three to five months significantly improves your chances of putting your type 2 diabetes into remission.

Research funded by an American company also found that some people with type 2 diabetes who followed a program that included a low-carb eating plan were in remission after two years. Participants in the study were supported to restrict their intake of carbs, initially to less than 30g per day and then gradually increasing the amount, based on personal tolerance and health goals.

If you have obesity, finding a way to lose weight can also reduce your risk of complications. There are different ways of doing this, and a low-carb diet is one option.

However, there's no evidence that following a low-carb diet is more beneficial in managing diabetes than other approaches in the long term, including a healthy, balanced diet. Research suggests that the best type of diet is one that you can maintain in the long term, so it's important to talk to your healthcare professional about what you think will work for you. Another option is the Mediterranean diet, which is also linked to reducing the risk of heart diseases and stroke.

WHAT TO CONSIDER BEFORE FOLLOWING A LOW-CARB DIET

If you treat your diabetes with insulin or any other medication that puts you at risk of hypos (low blood sugar levels), following a low-carb diet may increase this risk. Speak to your healthcare team about this so they can help you adjust your medications to reduce your risk of hypos. Your team may also support you to check your blood sugar levels more often.

Depending on the approach, following a low-carb diet may also lead to other side effects, such as constipation or bad breath. Although these can be unpleasant, they are usually temporary and shouldn't be harmful in the long term. Speak to your healthcare professional if you're concerned about any of these.

It's essential to first reduce your carb intake from unhealthy sources such as sugary drinks, pizzas, cakes, biscuits, chips, white bread, fruit juices, and smoothies. And it is a good idea to get your limited carbs from healthy high-fiber carb foods, such as pulses, nuts, vegetables, whole fruits, and whole grains, as well as unsweetened milk and Yogurt.

DIABETES: BEST DIETS FOR WEIGHT LOSS

For people with diabetes, reaching and maintaining a healthy weight is essential. A healthy weight helps manage blood sugar levels and reduce the chances of additional complications, such as a stroke or heart attack.

People with diabetes who want to lose weight must do so safely. Trying to lose weight too fast or being too restrictive can also lead to blood sugar levels. Obesity is a risk factor for type 2 diabetes. It is also becoming more common in people with type 1 diabetes.

A person with diabetes must consider several factors when deciding on the best way to lose weight. Factors to consider include their age, general health, and how much weight they have to lose. It is best to talk to a healthcare professional before starting any new weight-loss plan.

The best weight-loss diet for someone with diabetes is one they will stick to long-term. The following diets involve making beneficial long-term changes to help a person lose weight safely:

Mediterranean Diet

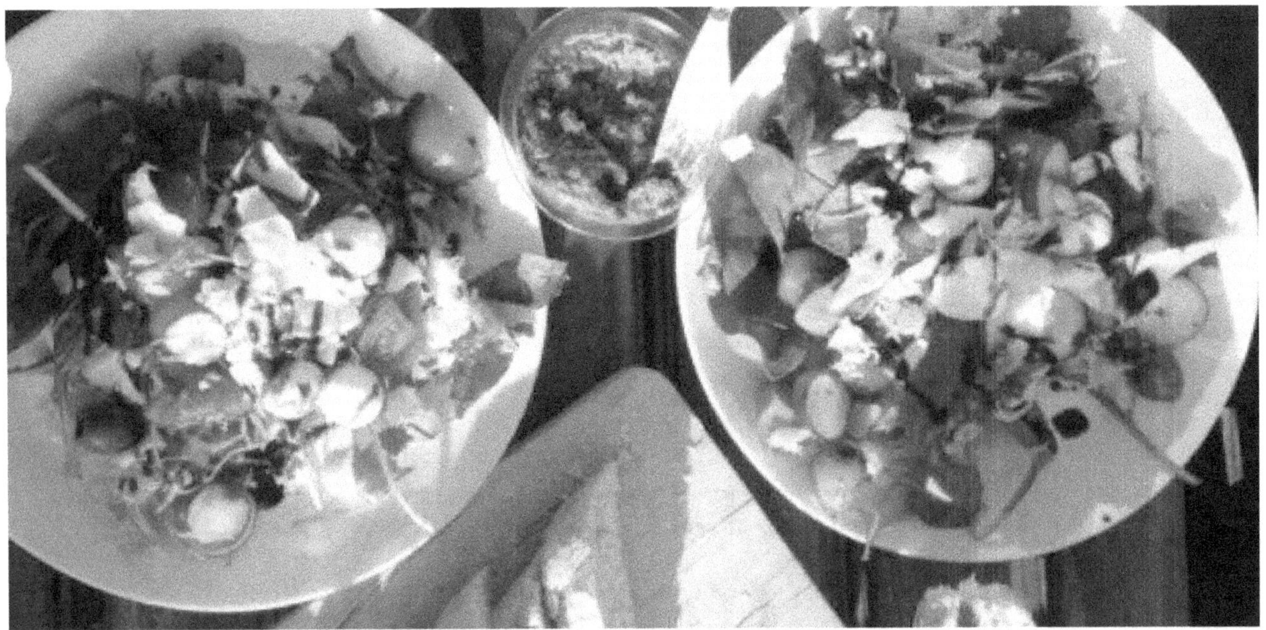

The Mediterranean diet involves food choices and cooking styles typical of some places in the Mediterranean region.

The diet includes:

- ☐ Plenty Of Vegetables
- ☐ Whole Grains
- ☐ Fruits In Moderation
- ☐ Nuts And Seeds

- ☐ Herbs And Spices
- ☐ Olive Oil
- ☐ Fish
- ☐ Eggs

The authors of a 2017 review noted that the Mediterranean diet might be a useful approach to weight loss for people with diabetes.

They highlighted a 2-year study that involved 36 adults with obesity and types 2 diabetes. The participants ate either a low-carbohydrate diet, a Mediterranean diet, or a low-fat diet for two years.

The Mediterranean diet was the most favorable for changes in insulin and fasting glucose levels. Those following the Mediterranean diet also lost an average of 1.5 kilograms (kg), or 3.3 pounds more than those on a low-fat diet.

Low-Carb Diet

Low-carb diets are a popular weight loss plan. Typically, low-carb diets limit a person's carbohydrate intake and include higher amounts of protein and healthful fats.

Examples of foods that to avoid on a low-carb diet include:

- ☐ Potatoes
- ☐ Rice
- ☐ White Bread
- ☐ Cakes
- ☐ Sweets
- ☐ Bagels
- ☐ Pasta

People on a low-carb diet should eat plenty of vegetables and get lots of protein from fish, lean meats, and eggs. To learn more about what to eat on a low-carb diet.Some studies show that low-carb diets may be effective and safe for people who have diabetes.

One study involved adults who had prediabetes or type 2 diabetes and had a body mass index (BMI) over 25.

The study participants ate either a very low-carb, high-fat, non-calorie restriction diet, a medium-carb, low-fat, calorie-restricted diet.

After three months, the group on the low-carb, high-fat diet lost 5.5 kg (about 12 pounds), compared to a 2.6 kg (5.7 pounds) weight loss for those following the medium-carb low-fat diet.

Additionally, 44% of those on the low-carb diet discontinued at least one diabetes medication.

It is vital to realize that there are different versions of low-carb diets. Some diets restrict carbohydrates to as low as 20 grams (g) or less per day, which may not be suitable for everyone.

Paleolithic Diet

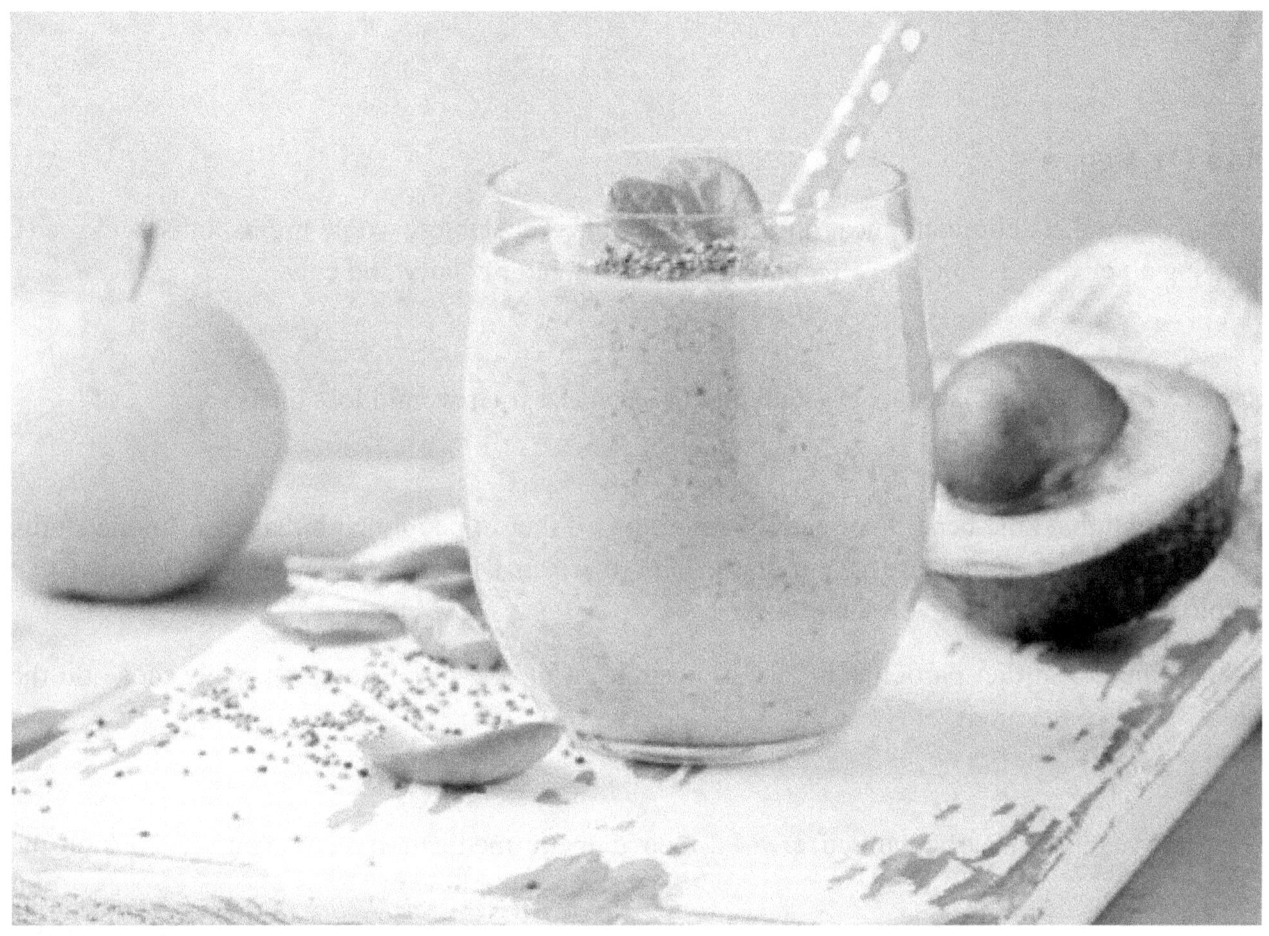

Fruits and vegetables are an everyday staple of weight-loss diets.

The Paleolithic or "paleo" diet attempts to replicate the diet that people ate thousands of years ago when hunting for food. Staples of a paleolithic diet include fruits, vegetables, lean meat, and fish.

Many of the foods included in the paleo diet are similar to those in a low-carb diet, as a paleo diet prohibits most grains' consumption.

In a small 2013 study, 13 people with type 2 diabetes followed the paleo diet for three months, then switched to a diabetic diet for three months.

The diabetic diet included evenly distributed meals that contained dietary FiberFiber, whole grain bread, cereals, and vegetables. The researchers found that the paleo diet was more filling per calorie than the diabetic diet. Participants noticed greater weight loss with the paleo diet but found it more challenging to sustain.

Vegetarian Or Vegan

Vegetarian and vegan diets eliminate meat and focus on fruits, vegetables, whole grains, nuts, and seeds. People following a vegan diet eliminate all animal products, including dairy and eggs.

A vegetarian or vegan diet may help people with diabetes achieve their weight loss goals.

A 2017 review highlighted the benefits of eating a plant-based diet in people with diabetes. In one study, 99 people of varying ages ate either a vegan diet or an American Diabetic Association (ADA) diet that included whole grains, fruits, vegetables, and meat.

After 22 weeks, the vegan diet participants lost an average of 6.5 kg (14.3 pounds), while those on the ADA diet lost 3.1 kg (6.8 pounds).

Also, 43% of the vegan diet participants decreased their diabetic medications, compared to 26% on the ADA diet.

5-DAY DIABETES MEAL PLAN FOR WEIGHT LOSS

Lose weight and keep your blood sugar steady with this healthy 5-day diabetes diet meal plan. Each of the five days offers healthy meals and snacks balanced for carbohydrates, protein, and FiberFiber to help keep your blood sugar steady as you cut calories to lose weight. Each meal contains 2-3 carb servings (30-45 grams of carbohydrates), and each snack is around 1 carb serving (15 grams of carbohydrates). Aim to keep your daily calorie total at 1,500 calories, which will put you on track to lose a healthy 1 to 2 pounds per week. We kept the days in this plan slightly under 1,500 calories so you'd have the freedom to add in a beverage of your choice or a diabetes-friendly dessert. And don't forget to stay hydrated! Aim for 64 oz. of water every day. With the healthy meals and snacks in this plan, losing weight with diabetes is a delicious and straightforward endeavor.

DAY 1

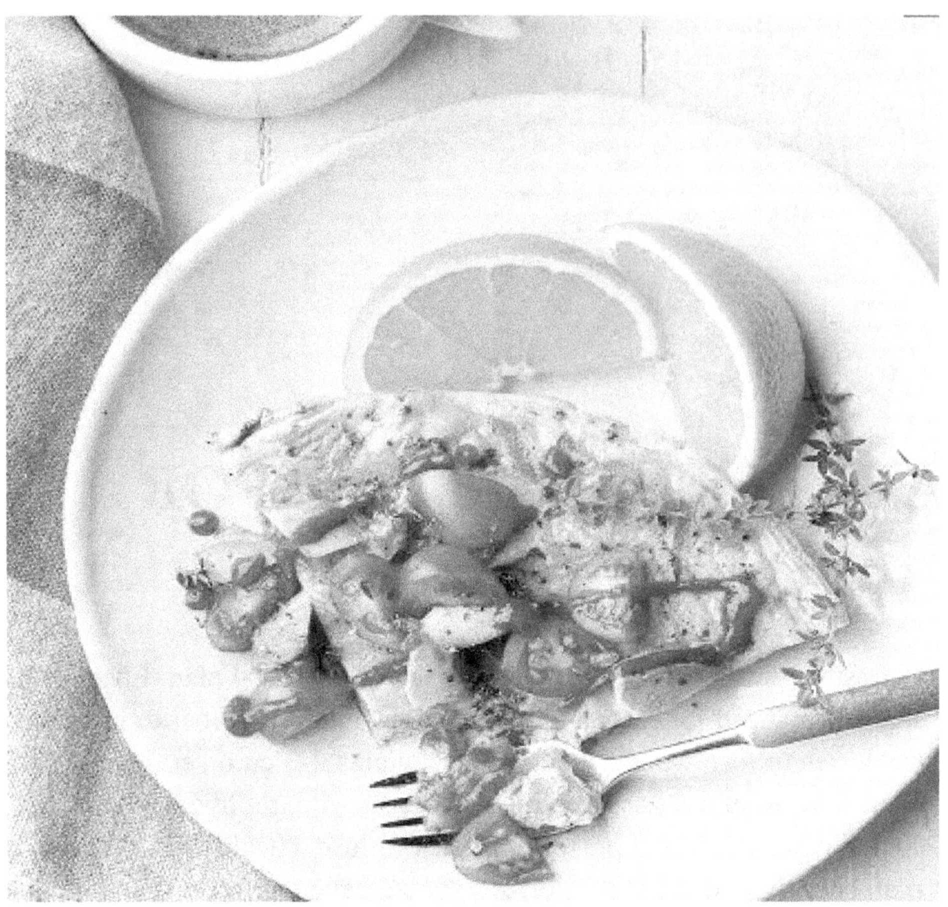

Breakfast

- ☐ 1 serving rainbow Frittata
- ☐ 1 slice whole-wheat toast
- ☐ 1 Tbsp. reduced-sugar jelly

Snack

- ☐ 1 medium banana
- ☐ 1 Tbsp. peanut butter

Lunch

7. 1 serving Spicy Thai Noodles

Snack

- ☐ 1 low-fat cheese stick
- ☐ 1 cup raspberries

Dinner

6. 1 serving Greek Chicken with Roasted Spring Vegetables

Daily Total: 1,359 calories, 136 g carbohydrates

DAY 2

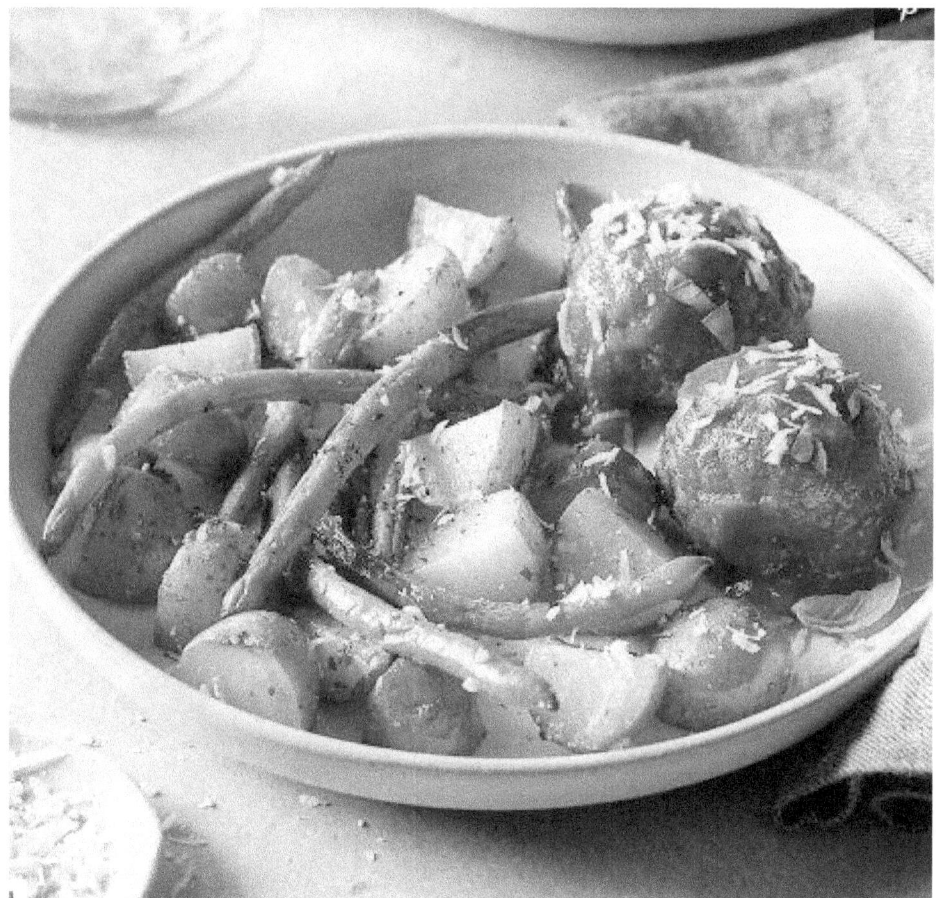

Breakfast

- [ ] 1 whole-wheat English muffin half
- [ ] 1/4 avocado, mashed
- [ ] 1 over-easy egg
- [ ] 1/2 cup grapes

Snack

- ☐ 2 Tbsp. raisins
- ☐ 2 Tbsp. unsalted peanuts

Lunch

- ☐ 1 serving Strawberry Arugula Salad
- ☐ 6 oz. light vanilla Greek Yogurt

Snack

8. 1/4 cup hummus
9. 1 cup carrot sticks

Dinner

- ☐ 1 serving Meatballs with Roasted Green Beans and Potatoes
- ☐ 1 cup raspberries

Daily Total: 1,244 calories, 146 g carbohydrates

DAY 3

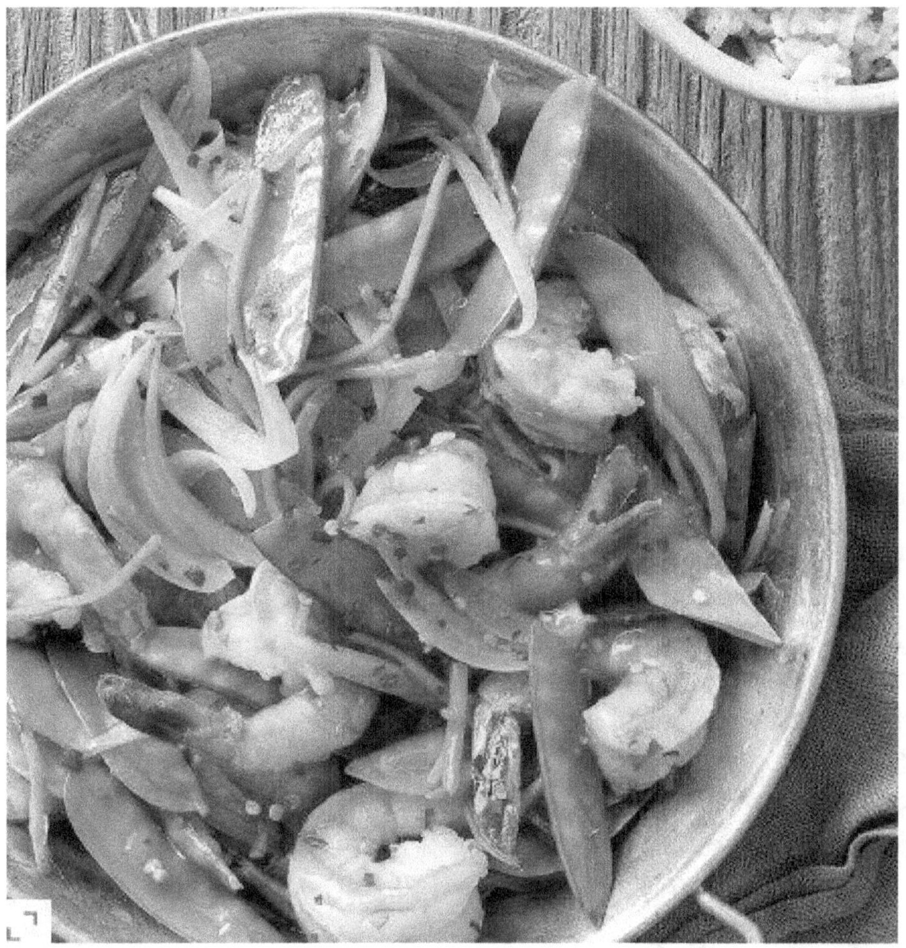

Breakfast

13. 1 hard-cooked egg

14. 1 serving Cherry-Mocha Smoothie

Snack

- ☐ 1 wedge light Swiss spreadable cheese

- ☐ 7 reduced-fat wheat crackers

- ☐ 1/2 cup grapes

Lunch

- ☐ 1 servingSpringtime Cacio e Pepe

- ☐ 1 cup carrot sticks

- ☐ 1 Tbsp. light ranch dressing

Snack

6. 2 Tbsp. raisins
7. 2 Tbsp. unsalted peanuts

Dinner

- [ ] 1 serving Shrimp and Pea Pod Stir-Fry
- [ ] 1 cup whole strawberries

Daily Total: 1,336 calories, 160 g carbohydrates

DAY 4

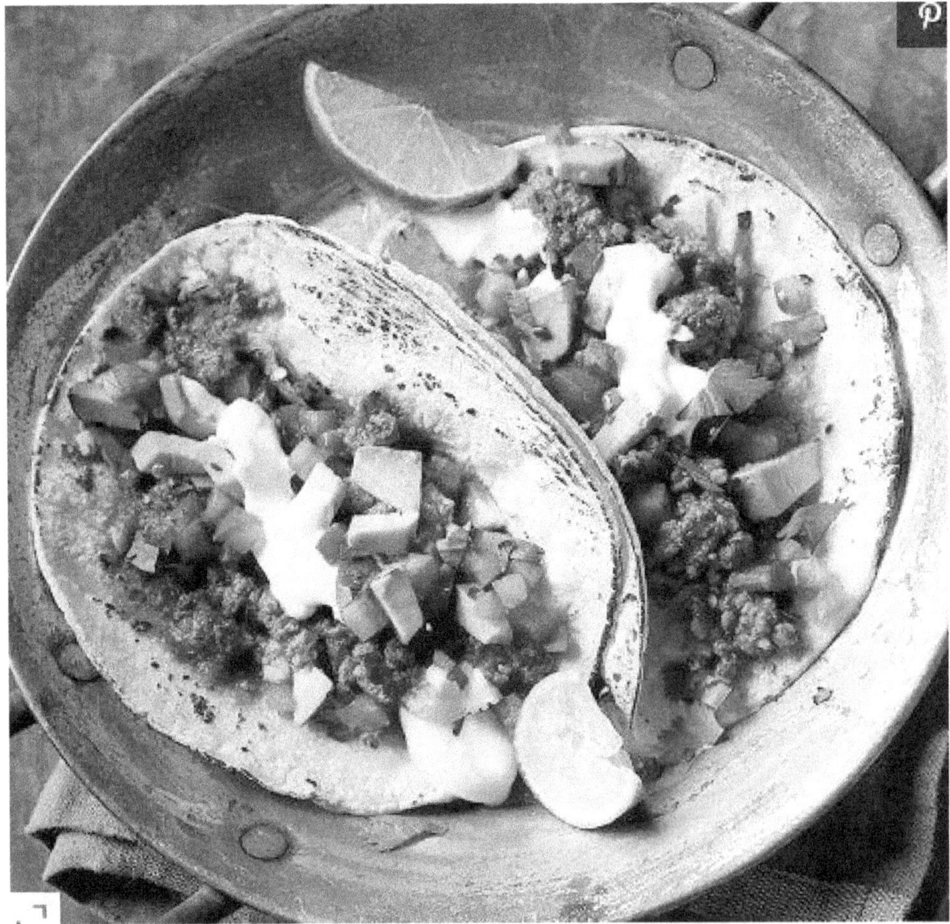

Breakfast

- [ ] 1 whole-wheat English muffin half

- ☐ 1/4 avocado, mashed
- ☐ 1 over-easy egg
- ☐ 1/2 cup grapes

Snack

- ☐ 1 cup carrot sticks
- ☐ 1 Tbsp. light ranch dressing

Lunch

- ☐ 1 serving Thai-Style Salad
- ☐ 1 medium banana

Snack

6. 1/4 cup hummus
7. 1 cup green bell pepper strips

Dinner

- ☐ 1 serving Chipotle Beef Tacos
- ☐ 1 serving Mexican Street Corn
- ☐ 1 serving Tangy Pepper Salad

Daily Total: 1,389 calories, 162 g carbohydrates

DAY 5

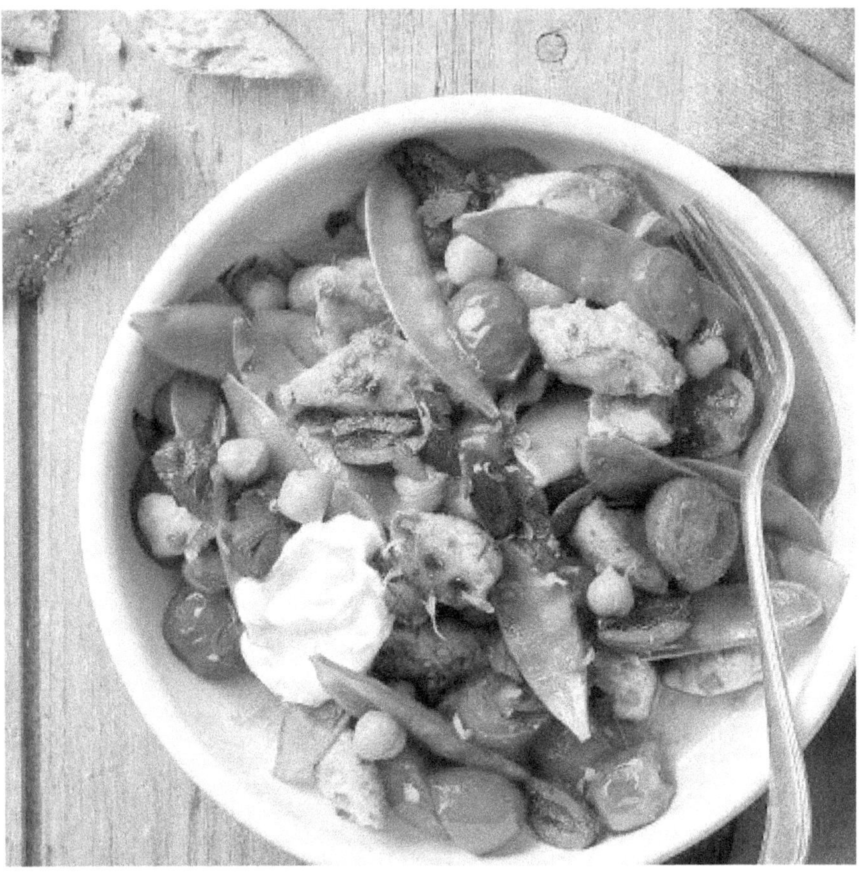

Breakfast

10. 1 cup oatmeal (prepared with water)

11. 1 Tbsp. peanut butter

12. 1/2 cup blueberries

Snack

- ☐ 1 cup grapes
- ☐ 1 low-fat mozzarella cheese stick

Lunch

- ☐ 1 serving Bacon Ranch Salad
- ☐ 1 cup whole strawberries

Snack

- ☐ 2 Tbsp. raisins
- ☐ 2 Tbsp. unsalted peanuts

Dinner

- ☐ 1 serving Spicy Chicken and Snow Pea Skillet
- ☐ 1 cup raspberries

Daily Total: 1,288 calories, 142 g carbohydrates

DIABETIC COOKING COOKBOOK

Finding tasty diabetes recipes can be challenging. This Diabetes Cookbook provides delicious recipes for cooking .

CONDIMENTS

Basil Pesto

a. 1 cup basil

b. 1/3 cup cashews

c. 2 garlic cloves, chopped

d. 1/2 cup olive oil or avocado oil Process basil, cashews, and garlic until smooth.

☐ Add oil in a slow stream. The process to combine.

☐ Transfer to a bowl.

☐ Season with salt and pepper.

☐ Stir to combine.

Allergies: SF, GF, DF, EF, V

Cilantro Pesto

☐ 1 cup cilantro

☐ 1/3 cup cashews

☐ 2 garlic cloves, chopped

☐ 1/2 cup olive oil or avocado oil Process cilantro, cashews, and garlic.

☐ Add oil in a slow stream. The process to combine.
☐ Transfer to a bowl.

□ Season with salt and pepper.

□ Stir to combine.

Allergies: SF, GF, DF, EF, V

Sundried Tomato Pesto

11. 3/4 cup sundried tomatoes

12. 1/3 cup cashews

13. 2 garlic cloves, chopped

14. 1/2 cup olive oil or cumin oil Process tomato, cashews, and garlic.

□ Add oil in a slow stream. The process to combine.

□ Transfer to a bowl.

□ Season with salt and pepper.

□ Stir to combine.

Allergies: SF, GF, DF, EF, V

BROTHS

Some recipes re□uire a cup or more of various broths, vegetables, Beef, or chicken broth. I usually cook the whole pot and freeze it.

Vegetable broth

Servings: 6 cups Ingredients

7. 1 tbsp. coconut oil
8. 1 large onion
9. 2 stalks celery, including some leaves
10. 2 large carrots
11. 1 bunch green onions, chopped
12. 8 cloves garlic, minced
13. 8 sprigs fresh parsley
14. 6 sprigs fresh thyme
15. 2 bay leaves
16. 1 tsp. salt
17. 2 □uarts of water

Allergies: SF, GF, DF, EF, V, NF

Instructions

□ Chop veggies into small chunks.

☐ Heat oil in a soup pot and add onion, scallions, celery, carrots, garlic, parsley, thyme, and bay leaves.

☐ Cook over high heat for 5 to 7 minutes, stirring occasionally.

☐ Bring to a boil and add salt.

☐ Lower heat and simmer, uncovered, for 30 minutes. Strain.

☐ Other ingredients to consider: broccoli stalk, celery root

Chicken Broth

Ingredients

☐ 4 lbs. fresh ChickenChicken (wings, necks, backs, legs, bones)

☐ 2 peeled onions or 1 cup chopped leeks

☐ 2 celery stalks

☐ 1 carrot

☐ 8 black peppercorns

☐ 2 sprigs fresh thyme

☐ 2 sprigs fresh parsley

☐ 1 tsp. salt Instructions –

Allergies: SF, GF, DF, EF, NF

7. Put cold water in a stockpot and add ChickenChicken.

8. Bring just to a boil.

9. Skim any foam from the surface.

10. Add other ingredients, return just to a boil, and reduce heat to a slow simmer.

11. Simmer for 2 hours.

12. Let cool to warm room temperature and strain.

13. Keep chilled and use or freeze broth within a few days.

14. Before using, defrost, and boil.

Beef Broth

Ingredients

- 4-5 pounds beef bones and few veal bones
- 1 pound of stew meat (chuck or flank steak) cut into 2-inch chunks
- Olive oil
- 1-2 medium onions, peeled and quartered
- 1-2 large carrots, cut into 1-2 inch segments 1 celery rib, cut into 1-inch segments
- 2-3 cloves of garlic, unpeeled
- Handful of parsley stems and leaves
- 1-2 bay leaves
- 10 peppercorns

Allergies: SF, GF, DF, EF, NF

Instructions -

- Heat oven to 375°F. Rub olive oil over the stew meat pieces, carrots, and onions.
- Place stew meat or beef scraps, stock bones, carrots, and onions in a large roasting pan.
- Roast in the oven for about 45 minutes, turning everything halfway through the cooking.
- Place everything from the oven in a large stockpot.
- Pour some boiling water in the oven pan and scrape up all of the browned bits, and pour all in the stockpot.
- Add parsley, celery, garlic, bay leaves, and peppercorns to the pot.
- Fill the pot with cold water to 1 inch over the top of the bones.
- Bring the stockpot to a steady simmer and then reduce the heat to low, so it just barely simmers.
- Cover the pot loosely and let simmer low and slow for 3-4 hours.
- Scoop away the fat and any scum that rises to the surface once in a while.
- After cooking, remove the bones and vegetables from the pot. Strain the broth.
- Let cool to room temperature and then put in the refrigerator.

☐ The fat will solidify once the broth has chilled. Discard the fat (or reuse it) and pour the broth into a jar and freeze it.

PASTES

Curry Paste

This should not be prepared in advance, but several curry recipes are using curry paste, and I decided to make the curry paste recipe out and have it separately.

When you see that the recipe uses curry paste, please go to this part of the book and prepare it from scratch.

Don't use processed curry pastes or curry powder; make it every time from scratch. Keep the original form(seeds, pods), ground them just before making the curry paste. You can dry heat in the skillet cloves, cardamom, cumin, and coriander and then crush them coarsely with mortar and pestle.

Ingredients

9. 2 onions, minced

10. 2 cloves garlic, minced

11. 2 teaspoons fresh ginger root, finely chopped

12. 6 whole cloves

13. 2 cardamom pods

14. 2 (2 inch) pieces cinnamon sticks, crushed

15. 1 tsp. ground cumin

16. 1 tsp. ground coriander

17. 1 tsp. salt

18. 1 tsp. ground cayenne pepper

19. 1 tsp. ground turmeric

Allergies: SF, GF, DF, EF, V, NF

Instructions -

- Heat oil in a frying pan over medium heat and fry onions until transparent.
- Stir in garlic, cumin, ginger, cloves, cinnamon, coriander, salt, cayenne, and turmeric.
- Cook for 1 minute over medium heat, stirring constantly.
- At this point, other curry ingredients should be added.

Tomato paste

Some recipes (chili) require tomato paste. I usually prepare 20 or so liters at once (when the tomato is in season, which is usually September) and freeze it.

Ingredients

- 5 lbs. chopped plump tomatoes
- 1/4 cup extra-virgin olive oil or avocado oil plus 2 tbsp.
- salt, to taste

Allergies: SF, GF, DF, EF, V, NF

Instructions –

- Heat 1/4 cup of the oil in a skillet over medium heat.
- Add tomatoes.
- Season with salt. Bring to a boil.
- Cook, stirring, until very soft, about 8 minutes.
- Pass the tomatoes through the most pleasing plate of a food mill.
- Push as much of the pulp through the sieve as possible and leave the seeds behind.

- ☐ Bring it to boil, lower it and then boil uncovered so that the liquid will thicken (approx. 30-40 minutes). That will give you homemade tomato juice.

- ☐ You get tomato paste if you boil for 60 minutes; it gets thick like store-bought ketchup.

- ☐ Store sealed in an airtight container in the refrigerator for up to one month, or freeze for up to 6 months.

Precooked beans

Some recipes also require that you cook some beans (butter beans, red kidney, garbanzo) in advance. Cooking beans takes around 3 hours, and it can be done in advance or every few weeks, and the rest gets frozen. Soak beans for 24 hours before cooking them. After the first boil, throw the water, add new water, and continue cooking. Some beans or lentils can be sprouted a few days before cooking, helping people with stomach problems.

BREAKFAST - OATMEAL

Oatmeal Breakfast

Allergies: SF, GF, DF, EF, V, NF

- ☐ 1/2 cup dry oatmeal
- ☐ 2 tsp. Of ground flax seeds
- ☐ 2 tsp. of sunflower seeds
- ☐ A dash of cinnamon
- ☐ 1 tsp. of cocoa

15. Cook oatmeal with hot water, and after that, mix all ingredients.

16. Sweeten if you have to with few drops of lucuma powder.

17. **Optional:** You can replace sunflower seeds with pumpkin seeds or chia seeds.

18. You can add a handful of blueberries or any berries instead of cocoa.

Oatmeal Yogurt Breakfast

Allergies: SF, GF, EF, NF

- [ ] 1/2 cup dry oatmeal
- [ ] Handful of blueberries (optional)
- [ ] 1 cups of low-fat Yogurt

Mix all ingredients and wait 20 minutes or leave overnight in the fridge if using steel cut oats

Cocoa Oatmeal

Allergies: SF, GF, DF, NF

Ingredients

- [ ] 1/2 cup dry oats
- [ ] 1 cup of water
- [ ] A pinch tsp. salt
- [ ] 1/2 tsp. ground vanilla bean
- [ ] 1 tbsp. cocoa powder
- [ ] 1 tbsp. lucuma powder
- [ ] 3 tbsp. ground flax seeds meal
- [ ] a dash of cinnamon
- [ ] 2 egg whites

Instructions

10. In a saucepan over high heat, place the oats and salt.

11. Cover with water.

12. Bring to a boil and cook for 3-5 minutes, stirring occasionally.

13. Keep adding 1/2 cup water if necessary as the mixture thickens.

14. In a separate bowl, whisk 4 tbsp. Water into the 1 tbsp. Cocoa powder to form a smooth sauce.

15. Add the vanilla to the pan and stir.

16. Turn the heat down to Low.

17. Add the egg whites and whisk immediately.

18. Add the flax meal and cinnamon.

19. Stir to combine.

20. Remove from heat, add lucuma powder, and serve immediately.

21. Topping suggestions: sliced strawberries, blueberries, or a few almonds.

Flax and Blueberry Vanilla Overnight Oats

Allergies: SF, GF, EF, V, NF

Ingredients –

- ☐ 1/2 cup dry oats
- ☐ 1/3 cup water
- ☐ 1/2 cup low-fat Yogurt
- ☐ 1/2 tsp. Ground vanilla bean
- ☐ 2 tbsp. flax seeds meal
- ☐ A pinch of salt
- ☐ Blueberries, almonds, blackberries, lucuma powder for topping

Instructions

9. Add the ingredients (except for toppings) to the bowl in the evening.

10. Refrigerate overnight.

11. In the morning, stir up the mixture.

12. It should be thick.

13. Add the toppings of your choice.

Apple Oatmeal

Allergies: SF, GF, DF, EF, V, NF

Ingredients -

- [ ] 1/2 grated apple
- [ ] 1/2 cup dry oats
- [ ] 1 cups water
- [ ] Dash of cinnamon
- [ ] 1 tsp. lucuma powder Instructions

- [ ] Cook the oats with the water for 3-5 minutes.
- [ ] Add grated apple and cinnamon.
- [ ] Stir in the lucuma powder.

Coconut Pomegranate Oatmeal

Allergies: SF, GF, DF, EF, V, NF

Ingredients -

7. 1/2 cup dry oats
8. 1/3 cup coconut milk
9. 1 cups water
10. 2 tbs. shredded unsweetened coconut
11. 1 tbs. flax seeds meal

12. 1 tbs. lucuma powder

13. 4 tbs. pomegranate seeds

Instructions

- ☐ Cook oats with coconut milk, water, and salt.
- ☐ Stir in the coconut, lucuma powder, and flaxseed meal.
- ☐ Sprinkle with extra coconut and pomegranate seeds.

SAVORY BREAKFASTS

Omelet with Leeks

Allergies: SF, GF, DF, NF

Cook 1 cup chopped leeks in little coconut oil until they get soft, and then mix the 2 beaten eggs.

Egg pizza crust

Allergies: SF, GF, DF, NF

Ingredients -

- ☐ 2 eggs
- ☐ 1/4 cup of coconut flour
- ☐ 1/2 cup of coconut milk
- ☐ 1 small crushed garlic clove

4. Mix and make an omelet.

Omelet with veggies

Allergies: SF, GF, DF, NF

Ingredients -

- ☐ 2 large eggs
- ☐ Salt
- ☐ Ground black pepper
- ☐ 1 tsp. olive oil or cumin oil
- ☐ 1cups spinach, cherry tomatoes, and 1 spoon of yogurt cheese
- ☐ Crushed red

☐ pepper flakes and a pinch of dill (optional)

Instructions

- ☐ Whisk 2 large eggs in a bowl.
- ☐ Season with salt and ground black pepper and set aside.
- ☐ Heat 1 tsp. Olive oil in a medium skillet over medium heat.
- ☐ Add baby spinach, tomatoes, cheese, and cook, tossing, until wilted (approx. 1 minute).
- ☐ Add eggs; cook, occasionally stirring, until just set, about 1 minute.
- ☐ Stir in cheese.
- ☐ Sprinkle with crushed red pepper flakes and dill.

Egg Muffins

Allergies: SF, GF, DF, NF

Serving: 4 muffins

Ingredients -

6. 4 eggs
7. 1/2 cup diced green bell pepper
8. 1/2 cup diced onion
9. 1/2 cup Spinach
10. 1/4 tsp. salt
11. 1/8 tsp. ground black pepper
12. 2 tbsp. water

Instructions

- ☐ Heat the oven to 350 degrees F. Oil 4 muffin cups.

☐ Beat eggs together.

☐ Mix in bell pepper, Spinach, onion, salt, black pepper, and water.

☐ Pour the mixture into muffin cups.

☐ Bake in the oven until muffins are done in the middle.

Smoked Salmon Scrambled Eggs

Allergies: SF, GF, DF, NF

Ingredients -

☐ 1 tsp coconut oil

☐ 2 eggs

☐ 1 Tbs water

☐ 2 oz smoked salmon, sliced

☐ 1/4 avocado

☐ ground black pepper, to taste

☐ 2 chives, minced (or use 1 green onion, thinly sliced)

Instructions

☐ Heat a skillet over medium heat.

☐ Add coconut oil to the pan when hot.

☐ Meanwhile, scramble eggs.

☐ Add eggs to the hot skillet, along with smoked salmon.

☐ Stirring continuously, cook eggs until soft and fluffy.

☐ Remove from heat.

☐ Top with avocado, black pepper, and chives to serve.

Steak and Eggs

Allergies: SF, GF, DF, NF

Ingredients -

- ☐ 1/4 lb boneless beef steak or pork tenderloin • 1/4 tsp ground black pepper
- ☐ 1/4 tsp sea salt (optional)
- ☐ 1 tsp coconut oil
- ☐ 1/4 onion, diced
- ☐ 1/2 red bell pepper, diced
- ☐ 1 handful spinach or arugula
- ☐ 1 egg Instructions

- ☐ Season sliced steak or pork tenderloin with sea salt and black pepper.
- ☐ Heat a sauté pan over high heat.
- ☐ Add 1 tsp coconut oil, onions, and meat when the pan is hot, and sauté until the steak is slightly cooked.
- ☐ Add spinach and red bell pepper, and cook until steak is done to your liking.
- ☐ Meanwhile, heat a small frypan over medium heat.
- ☐ Add remaining coconut oil, and fry two eggs.
- ☐ Top steak with a fried egg to serve.

Egg Bake

Allergies: SF, GF, DF, NF

Ingredients -

5. 1/2 cup chopped red peppers or Spinach

6. 1/4 cup zucchini

7. 1/2 tbsp. coconut oil

8. 1/4 cup sliced green onions

9. 2 eggs

10. 1/4 cup coconut milk

11. 1/8 cup almond flour

12. 1 tbsp. Minced fresh parsley

13. 1/4 tsp. dried basil

14. 1/8 tsp. salt

15. 1/8 tsp. ground black pepper

Instructions

- Preheat oven to 350 degrees F.
- Put coconut oil in a skillet.
- Heat it to medium heat.
- Add mushrooms, onions, zucchini, and red pepper (or Spinach) until vegetables are tender, about 5 minutes.
- Drain veggies and spread them over the baking dish.
- Beat eggs in a bowl with milk, flour, parsley, basil, salt, and pepper.
- Pour egg mixture into baking dish.
- Bake in the preheated oven until the center is set (approx. 35 to 40 minutes).

Frittata

Allergies: SF, GF, DF, NF

Ingredients -

- ☐ 1 tbsp. olive oil or avocado oil
- ☐ 1/2 Zucchini, sliced
- ☐ 1/4 cup torn fresh Spinach
- ☐ 1 tbsp. sliced green onions
- ☐ 1/4 tsp. crushed garlic, salt, and pepper to taste
- ☐ 1/8 cup coconut milk
- ☐ 2 eggs Instructions

- ☐ Heat olive oil in a skillet over medium heat.
- ☐ Add zucchini and cook until tender.
- ☐ Mix in Spinach, green onions, and Garlic.
- ☐ Season with salt and pepper. Continue cooking until Spinach is wilted.
- ☐ In a separate bowl, beat together eggs and coconut milk.
- ☐ Pour into the skillet over the vegetables.
- ☐ Reduce heat to low, cover, and cook until eggs are firm (5 to 7 minutes).

Naan Pancakes Crepes

Allergies: SF, GF, DF, EF, V

Ingredients -

- ☐ 1/2 cup almond flour
- ☐ 1/2 cup Tapioca Flour
- ☐ 1 cup Coconut Milk
- ☐ Salt
- ☐ coconut oil

☐ Instructions

6. Mix all the ingredients.

7. Heat a pan over medium heat and pour batter to desired thickness.

8. Once the batter looks firm, flip it over to cook the other side.

9. If you want this to be a dessert crepe or pancake, then omit the salt.

10. You can add minced garlic or ginger in the batter if you want, or some spices.

Zucchini Pancakes

Allergies: SF, GF, DF

Ingredients -

- ☐ 1 small zucchini
- ☐ 1 tbsp. Chopped onion
- ☐ 2 beaten eggs
- ☐ 3 tbsp. Almond flour
- ☐ 1/2 tsp. salt
- ☐ 1/2 tsp. ground black pepper
- ☐ coconut oil

Instructions

- ☐ Heat the oven to 300 degrees F.
- ☐ Grate the zucchini into a bowl and stir in the onion and eggs.
- ☐ Stir in 6 tbsp. of the flour, salt, and pepper.
- ☐ Heat a large sauté pan over medium heat and add coconut oil to the pan.
- ☐ When the oil is hot, lower the heat to medium-low and add batter into the pan.
- ☐ Cook the pancakes for about 2 minutes on each side, until browned.
- ☐ Place the pancakes in the oven.

Smoothies

Put the li□uid in first. Surrounded by tea or Yogurt, the blender blades can move freely. Next, add chunks of fruits or vegetables. Leafy greens are going into the pitcher last. The preferred li□uid is green tea, but you can use almond or coconut milk or herbal tea.

Start slow. If your blender has sped, start it on Low to break up big pieces of fruit. Continue blending until you get a puree. If your blender can pulse, pulse a few times before switching to a puree mode. Once you have your li□uid and fruit pureed, start adding greens, very slowly. Wait until the previous batch of greens has been thoroughly blended.

Thicken? Added too much tea or coconut milk? Thicken your smoothie by adding ice cubes, flax meal, chia seeds, or oatmeal. Once you get used to smoothies' various tastes, add any seaweed, spirulina, chlorella powder, or ginger for an additional kick. Think of adding any nut butter or sesame paste too or some oils.

Rotate! Rotate your greens; don't always drink the same smoothie! In the beginning, try 2 different greens every week and later introduce the third and fourth one weekly. And keep rotating them. Don't use Spinach and Kale all the time.

Try beets greens; they have a pinch of pink in them, which adds great color to your smoothie. Here is the list of leafy green for you to try: Spinach, Kale, dandelion, chards, beet leaves, arugula, lettuce, collard greens, bok choy, cabbage, cilantro, parsley.

Flavor! Flavor smoothies with ground vanilla bean, cinnamon, lucuma powder, nutmeg, cloves, almond butter, cayenne pepper, ginger, or just about any seeds or chopped nuts combination.

Not only are green smoothies high in nutrients, vitamins, and fiber, they can also make any vegetable you probably don't like (be it kale, spinach, or broccoli) taste great.

The secret behind blending the perfect smoothie is using sweet fruits or nuts, or seeds to give your drink a uniＱue taste. There's a reason kale and spinach seem to be the main ingredients in almost every green smoothie.

Not only do they give smoothies their green color, but they are also packed with calcium, protein, and iron. Although blending alone increases the accessibility of carotenoids, since fats are known to increase carotenoid absorption from leafy greens, it is possible that coconut oil, nuts, and seeds in a smoothie could increase absorption further. If you can't find some ingredient, replace it with the closest one.

GREEN SMOOTHIES

Kale Kiwi Smoothie

- ☐ 1 cup Kale, chopped
- ☐ 1 Apple
- ☐ 2 Kiwis
- ☐ 1 tablespoon flax seeds
- ☐ 1 tablespoon lucuma powder
- ☐ 1 cup crushed ice

Zucchini Apples Smoothie

- 1/2 cup zucchini
- 1 Apple
- 3/4 avocado
- 1 stalk Celery
- 1 Lemon
- 1 tbsp. Spirulina
- 1 1/2 cups crushed ice

Dandelion Smoothie

3. 1 cup Dandelion greens
4. 1 cup Spinach
5. ½ cup tahini
6. 1 Red Radish
7. 1 tbsp. chia seeds
8. 1 cup lavender tea

Broccoli Apple Smoothie

- 1 Apple
- 1 cup Broccoli
- 1 tbsp. Cilantro
- 1 Celery stalk
- 1 cup crushed ice
- 1 tbsp. crushed Seaweed

Salad Smoothie

- ☐ 1 cup Spinach
- ☐ ½ cucumber
- ☐ 1/2 small onion
- ☐ 2 tablespoons Parsley
- ☐ 2 tablespoons lemon juice
- ☐ 1 cup crushed ice
- ☐ 1 tbsp. olive oil or cumin oil
- ☐ ¼ cup Wheatgrass

SALAD DRESSINGS

Italian Dressing

Allergies: SF, GF, DF, EF, V, NF

- ☐ 2 tsp. olive oil or avocado oil
- ☐ lemon

☐ minced garlic

☐ salt

Yogurt Dressing

Allergies: SF, GF, DF, EF, V, NF

3. 1 cup of plain low-fat Greek Yogurt or low-fat buttermilk

4. 1 tsp. olive oil or avocado oil

5. minced garlic

6. salt

7. lemon Occasionally, add a tsp. of mustard or some herbs like basil, oregano, marjoram, chives, thyme, parsley, dill, or mint.

If you like spicy hot food, add some cayenne to the Dressing. It will speed up your metabolism and have an interesting hot spicy effect in cold Yogurt or buttermilk.

SALADS

Large Fiber Loaded Salad with Italian Dressing

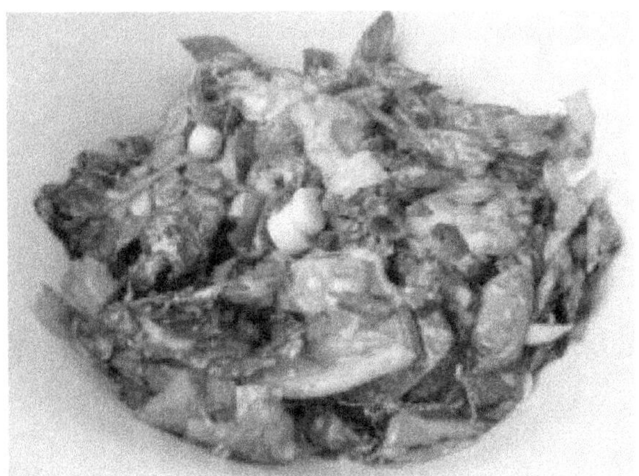

Allergies: SF, GF, EF, NF

- ☐ 2 cups of Spinach
- ☐ 1 cup of shredded cabbage, sauerkraut, or lettuce. Cabbage has more substance.
- ☐ Italian or Yogurt dressing
- ☐ Cayenne pepper (optional)
- ☐ Few sprigs of cilantro (optional)
- ☐ 2 spring (green) onions (optional)

Large Fiber Loaded Salad with Yogurt Dressing

Serves 1 - Allergies: SF, GF, EF, NF

- ☐ 2 cups of Spinach
- ☐ 1 cup of shredded cabbage or lettuce. Cabbage has more substance.
- ☐ Italian or Yogurt dressing
- ☐ Cayenne pepper (optional)
- ☐ Few sprigs of cilantro (optional)
- ☐ 2 spring (green) onions (optional

Large Fiber Loaded Salad as a meal on its own

Allergies: SF, GF, EF, NF

This is what I eat every second evening, and I can't get enough of it!!! This is the the real secret to lose weight while having a full stomach with grade A ingredients!!

7. 2 cups of Spinach
8. 2 cups of shredded cabbage
9. Yogurt dressing
10. Cayenne pepper (optional)
11. Few sprigs of cilantro (optional)
12. 3 spring (green) onions
13. 10 o.z. low-fat farmers' cheese

4. Pour yogurt dressing into the salad bowl.
5. Add farmers' cheese and mix thoroughly.
6. Cut spring onions in small pieces and add to the cheese mixture and mix.
7. Add Spinach and cabbage and mix thoroughly.
8. Add spices (optional).

Greek Salad

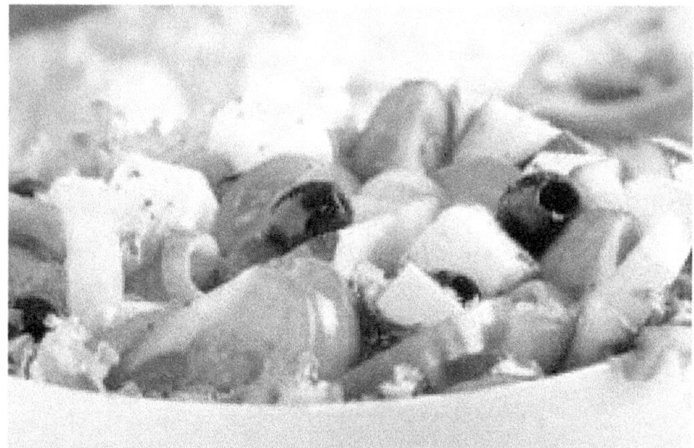

Allergies: SF, GF, EF, NF

- [ ] 1 head romaine lettuce
- [ ] 1/2 lb. plump tomatoes
- [ ] 3 oz. Greek or black olives, sliced
- [ ] 2 oz. sliced radishes
- [ ] 4 oz. low-fat feta or goat cheese
- [ ] 2 oz. anchovies (optional)

Dressing:

a. 2 oz. olive oil or avocado oil
b. 2 oz. fresh lemon juice
c. 1/2 tsp. dried oregano
d. 1/4 tsp. black pepper
e. 1/4 tsp. salt
f. 2 cloves garlic, minced

- [ ] Wash and cut lettuce into pieces. Slice tomatoes in quarters.
- [ ] Combine olives, lettuce, tomatoes, and radishes in a large bowl.
- [ ] Mix dressing ingredients and toss with vegetables.
- [ ] Pour out into a shallow serving bowl.
- [ ] Crumble feta/goat cheese overall, and arrange anchovy fillets on top (if desired).

Strawberry Spinach Salad

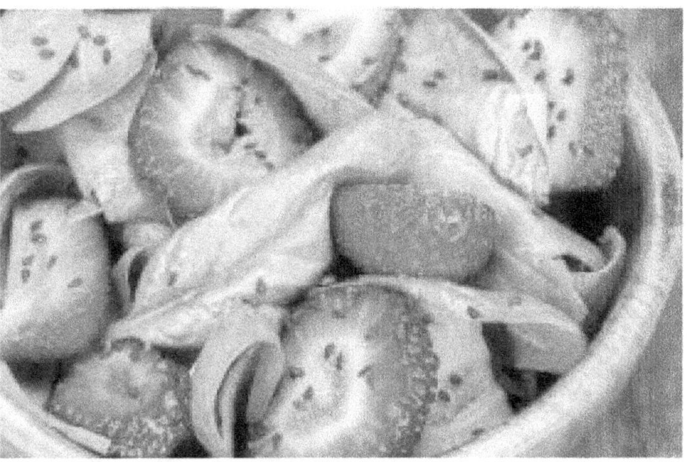

Allergies: SF, GF, DF, EF, V

Ingredients -

- ☐ 1 tbsp. black sesame seeds
- ☐ 1 tbsp. poppy seeds
- o 1/4 cup olive oil or cumin oil
- o 1/8 cup lemon juice
- o 1/8 tsp. paprika
- o 1/2 bag fresh spinach - chopped, washed, and dried
- o 1 cup strawberries, sliced
- o 1/4 cup toasted slivered almonds Instructions

☐ Whisk together the sesame seeds, olive oil, poppy seeds, paprika, lemon juice, and onion. Refrigerate.

☐ In a large bowl, combine the spinach, strawberries, and almonds.

☐ Pour dressing over salad.

☐ Toss and refrigerate 15 minutes before serving.

Cucumber, Cilantro, Quinoa Tabbouleh

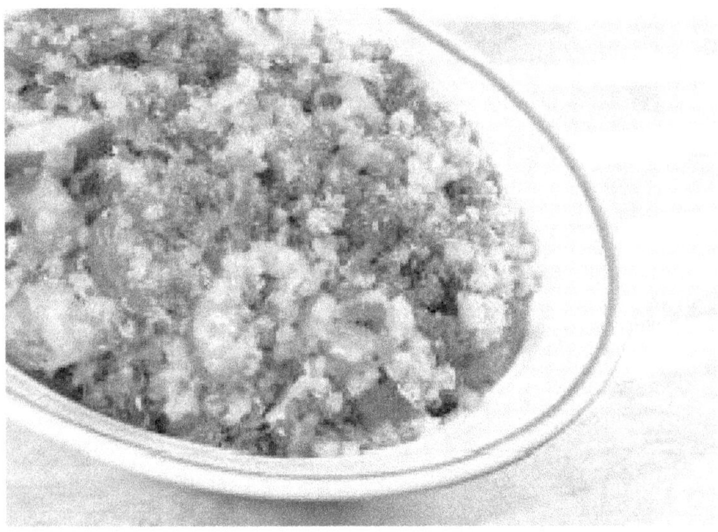

Serves 2

Allergies: SF, GF, DF, EF, NF, V

Ingredients -

    a. 1/2 cup cooked ☐uinoa mixed with 1 tbsp. sesame seeds

    b. 1/2 cup chopped tomato and green pepper

    c. 1 cup chopped cucumber

    d. 1/2 cup chopped cilantro Dressing:

    e. 1 tbsp. olive oil or avocado oil

    f. 1 tbsp. fresh lemon juice

    g. pinch of black pepper

    h. pinch of sea salt

Instructions: Mix all ingredients.

Almond, Quinoa, Red Peppers & Arugula Salad

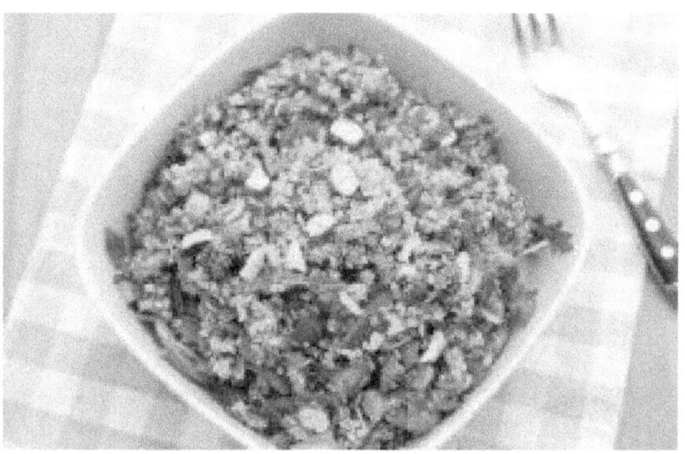

Serves 2

Allergies: SF, GF, DF, EF, NF, V

Ingredients -

- o   1/2 cup cooked ⬜uinoa mixed with 1 tbsp. pumpkin seeds
- o   1/2 cup chopped almonds
- o   1 cup chopped arugula
- o   1/2 cup sliced red peppers Dressing:
- o   1 tbsp. olive oil or cumin oil
- o   1 tbsp. fresh lemon juice
- o   pinch of black pepper
- o   pinch of sea salt

Instructions: Mix all ingredients.

Asparagus, Quinoa & Red Peppers Salad

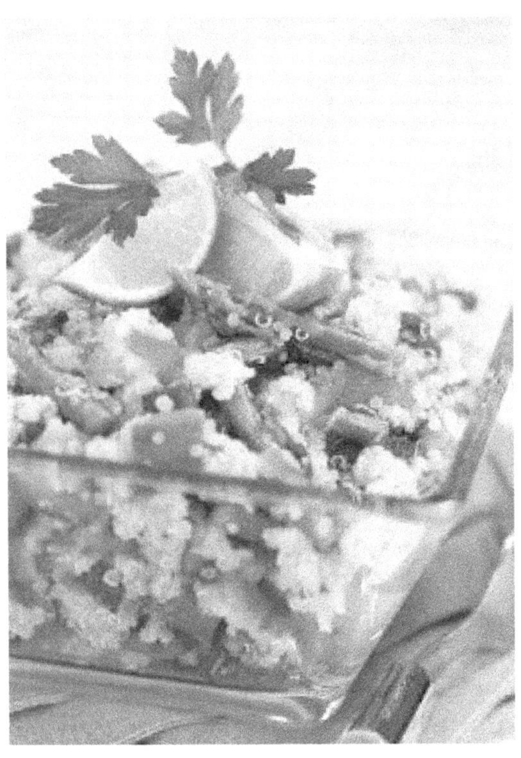

Serves 2

Allergies: SF, GF, DF, EF, NF, V

Ingredients –

- o   1/2 cup cooked □uinoa mixed with 1 tbsp. sunflower seeds
- o   1 cup sliced red peppers
- o   1 cup grilled asparagus
- o   Garnish with lime and parsley

Dressing:

a.   1 tbsp. olive oil or avocado oil

b.   1 tbsp. fresh lemon juice

c.   pinch of black pepper

d.   pinch of sea salt

Instructions: Mix all ingredients.

Chickpeas, Quinoa, Cucumber & Tomato Salad

Serves 2

Allergies: SF, GF, DF, EF, NF, V

Ingredients -

a. 1/2 cup cooked Quinoa mixed with 1 tbsp. sesame seeds
b. 1/2 cup cooked chickpeas
c. 1 cup chopped cucumber and green onions
d. 1/2 cup chopped tomato Dressing:
e. 1 tbsp. olive oil or avocado oil
f. 1 tbsp. fresh lemon juice
g. pinch of black pepper
h. pinch of sea salt

Instructions: Mix all ingredients

Quinoa Salad

Allergies: SF, GF, EF

Ingredients -

For the salad

o 1/2 cup cooked Quinoa
o 1/2 cup frozen green peas
o 1/4 cup low-fat feta cheese
o 4 oz. pork, cubed
o 1/8 cup freshly chopped basil and cilantro
o 1/8 cup almonds, pulsed in a food processor until crushed For the dressing
o 1/8 cup lemon juice (1 juicy lemon)

o   1/8 cup olive oil or cumin oil • 1/8 tsp. salt (more to taste)

Instructions

9. Bring a pot of water to boil, and then lower the heat.

10. Add the peas and cook covered until bright green. In the meantime, brown pork in a skillet.

11. Toss the ⬜uinoa with the pork, peas, feta, herbs, and almonds.

12. Puree all the dressing ingredients in the food processor.

13. Toss the Dressing with the salad ingredients.

14. Season generously with salt and pepper.

15. Serve tossed with fresh baby spinach.

Cauliflower & Eggs Salad

Allergies: SF, GF, NF

Ingredients -

o   1 cup chopped Cauliflower

o   2 hardboiled eggs - chopped,

o   2 oz. shredded cheddar cheese, low-fat

o   1/2 red onion, celery,

o   1 dill pickles,

o   1 tbsp. Yellow mustard.

Mix all ingredients.

Greek Cucumber Salad

Allergies: SF, GF, EF, NF

Ingredients -

o   2 cucumbers, sliced

o   1 teaspoon salt

o   2 tbsp. lemon juice

- o 1/4 tsp. paprika
- o 1/4 tsp. white pepper
- o 1/2 clove garlic, minced
- o 2 fresh green onions, diced
- o 1 cup thick Greek Yogurt
- o 1/4 tsp. paprika

Instructions

- ☐ Slice cucumbers thinly sprinkle with salt and mix.
- ☐ Set aside for one hour.
- ☐ Mix lemon juice, Water, garlic, paprika, and white pepper, and set aside.
- ☐ S☐ueeze li☐uid from cucumber slices a few at a time, and place slices in the bowl.
- ☐ Discard li☐uid.
- ☐ Add lemon juice mixture, green onions, and Yogurt.
- ☐ Mix and sprinkle additional paprika or dill over the top. Chill for 1-2 hours

Mediterranean Salad

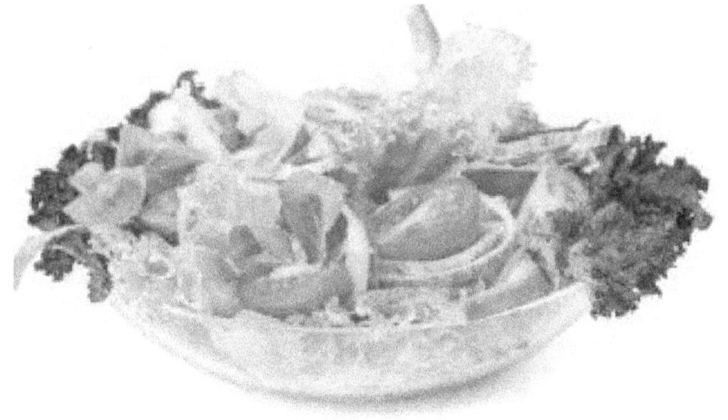

Allergies: SF, GF, DF, EF, V, NF

Ingredients -

   a.   1 small head romaine lettuce, torn
   b.   1 tomato, diced
   c.   1 small cucumber, sliced
   d.   1/2 green bell pepper, sliced
   e.   1/2 small onion, cut into rings
   f.   3 radishes, thinly sliced
   g.   1/4 cup flat-leaf parsley, chopped
   h.   1/4 cup olive oil or avocado oil
   i.   2 tbsp. lemon juice
   j.   1 garlic clove, minced
   k.   Salt & pepper
   l.   1 tsp. fresh mint, minced

Instructions

9. Combine lettuce, tomatoes, cucumber, pepper, onion, radishes & parsley in a salad bowl.
10. Whisk together olive oil, lemon juice, Garlic, salt, pepper & mint.
11. Pour over salad & toss to coat.

Apple Coleslaw

Allergies: SF, GF, DF, EF, V, NF

Ingredients -

   o   2 cups chopped cabbage (various color)
   o   1 tart apple chopped
   o   1 celery, chopped

- o 1 red pepper chopped
- o 4 tsp. olive oil or avocado oil
- o juice of 1 lemon
- o 1 Tbs. lucuma powder (optional)
- o dash sea salt

Instructions

- ☐ Toss the cabbage, apple, celery, and pepper together in a large bowl.
- ☐ In a smaller bowl, whisk the remaining ingredients.
- ☐ Drizzle over coleslaw and toss to coat.

Appetizers

Hummus

Allergies: SF, GF, DF, EF, V, NF

Ingredients -

- ☐ 1/2 cup cooked chickpeas (garbanzo beans)
- ☐ 1/2 small lemon
- ☐ 2 Tbsp. tahini
- ☐ Half of a garlic clove, minced
- ☐ 1 tbsp. olive oil or cumin oil, plus more for serving
- ☐ 1/2 tsp. salt
- ☐ 1/4 tsp. ground cumin
- o 2 to 3 tbsp. water
- o Dash of ground paprika for serving

Instructions

10. Combine tahini and lemon juice and blend for 1 minute.
11. Add the olive oil, minced garlic, cumin, and salt to the tahini and lemon mixture.
12. Process for 30 seconds, scrape sides, and then process 30 seconds more.
13. Add half of the chickpeas to the food processor and process for 1 minute.
14. Scrape sides, add remaining chickpeas, and process for 1 to 2 minutes.
15. Transfer the hummus into a bowl, then drizzle about 1 tbsp. of olive oil over the top and sprinkle with paprika.

Guacamole

Allergies: SF, GF, DF, EF, V, NF

Ingredients -

- o   2 ripe avocados
- o   2 tbsp. freshly squeezed lemon juice (1 lemon)
- o   4 dashes hot pepper sauce
- o   1/4 cup diced onion
- o   1 garlic clove, minced
- o   1/2 tsp. salt
- o   1/2 tsp. ground black pepper
- o   1 small tomato, seeded, and small-diced

Instructions

3. Cut the avocados in half, remove the pits, and scoop the flesh out.
4. Immediately add the lemon juice, hot pepper sauce, garlic, onion, salt, and pepper, and toss well.
5. Dice avocados. Add the tomatoes.
6. Mix well and taste for salt and pepper.

Baba Ghanoush

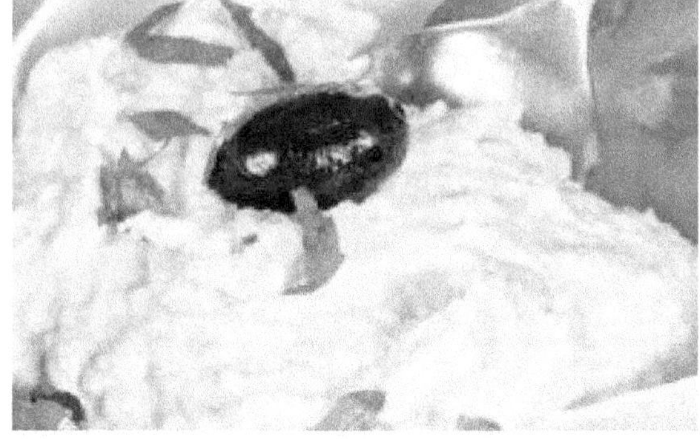

Allergies: SF, GF, DF, EF, V, NF

Ingredients –

a. 1 eggplant

b. 1/4 cup tahini, plus more as needed

c. 1 garlic clove, minced

d. 1/8 cup fresh lemon juice, plus more as needed

e. 1 pinch ground cumin

f. salt, to taste

g. 1 tbsp. Extra-virgin olive oil or avocado oil

h. 1 tbsp. chopped flat-leaf parsley

i. 1/4 cup brine-cured black olives, such as Kalamata

Instructions:

- ☐ Grill eggplant for 10 to 15 minutes. Heat the oven (375 F).
- ☐ Put the eggplant on a baking sheet and bake 15-20 minutes or until very soft.
- ☐ Remove from the oven, let cool, and peel off and discard the skin.
- ☐ Put the eggplant flesh in a bowl. Using a fork, mash the eggplant to a paste.
- ☐ Add the 1/4 cup tahini, garlic, cumin, 1/4 cup lemon juice and mix well.
- ☐ Season with salt to taste.
- ☐ Transfer the mixture to a serving bowl and spread with the back of a spoon to form a shallow well.
- ☐ Drizzle the olive oil over the top and sprinkle with the parsley.

Espinacase la Catalana

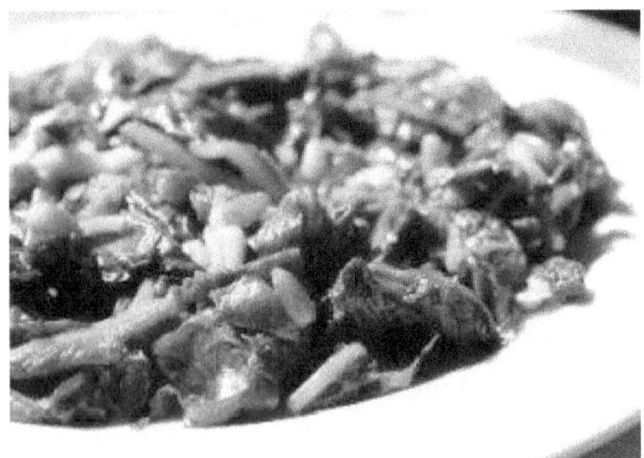

Allergies: SF, GF, DF, EF, V

    a. 1 cup Spinach

    b. 1 cloves garlic

    c. 2 tbsp cashews

    d. olive oil or avocado oil Instructions

Ingredients -

- ☐ Wash the Spinach and trim off the stems. Steam the Spinach for few minutes.
- ☐ Peel and slice the garlic.
- ☐ Pour a few tablespoons of olive oil and cover the bottom of a frying pan.
- ☐ Heat pan on medium and sauté garlic for 1-2 minutes.
- ☐ Add the cashews to the pan and continue to sauté for 1 minute.
- ☐ Add the Spinach and mix well, coating with oil.
- ☐ Salt to taste.
- ☐ Serve at room temperature.

Tapenade

Allergies: SF, GF, DF, EF, V, NF

Ingredients -

- o 1/4 pound olives with pit removed
- o 2 anchovy fillets, rinsed
- o 1 small clove garlic, minced
- o 2 tbsp. capers
- o 2 fresh basil leaves
- o 1 tbsp. freshly s☐ueezed lemon juice

o   1 tbsp. extra-virgin olive oil or cumin oil

Instructions

8. Rinse the olives in cold water.

9. Place all ingredients in the bowl of a food processor.

10. The process to combine until it becomes a coarse paste.

11. Transfer to a bowl and serve.

SOUPS

Cream of Broccoli Soup

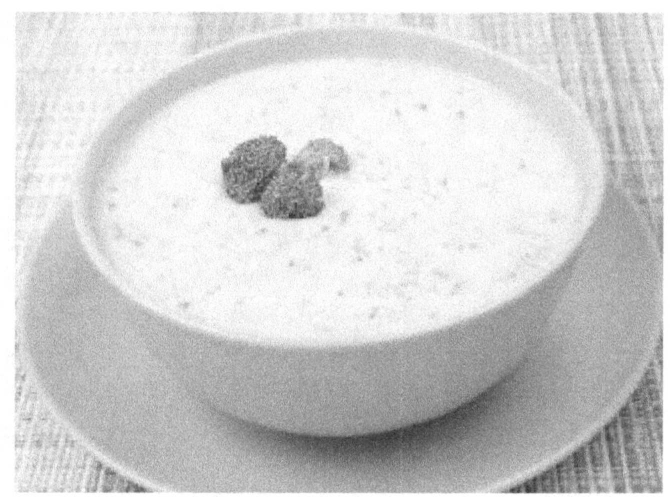

Allergies: SF, GF, EF, NF

Ingredients -

- o 1 pound broccoli, fresh
- o 1 cup of water
- o 1/4 tsp. salt, pepper to taste
- o 1/4 cup tapioca flour, mixed with 1 cup cold water
- o 1/4 cup coconut cream
- o 1/4 cup low-fat farmers' cheese Steam or boil Broccoli until it gets tender.

☐ Put 1 cup of water and coconut cream on top of a double boiler.

☐ Add salt, cheese, and pepper.

☐ Heat until cheese gets melted.

☐ Add Broccoli. Mix water and tapioca flour in a small bowl.

☐ Stir tapioca mixture into cheese mixture in double boiler and heat until soup thickens.

Lentil Soup

Allergies: SF, GF, DF, EF, NF

Ingredients -

- o 1 tbsp. olive oil or avocado oil
- o 1/2 cup finely chopped onion
- o 1/4 cup chopped carrot
- o 1/4 cup chopped celery
- o 1 teaspoons salt
- o 1/2 pound lentils
- o 1/2 cup chopped tomatoes
- o 1-☐uart chicken or vegetable broth
- o 1/4 tsp. ground coriander & toasted cumin

Instructions

7. Place the olive oil into a large Dutch oven.
8. Set over medium heat.
9. Once hot, add the celery, onion, carrot, and salt and do until the onions are translucent.
10. Add the lentils, tomatoes, cumin, broth, and coriander and stir to combine.
11. Increase the heat and bring just to a boil.
12. Reduce the heat, cover, and simmer at a low until the lentils are tender (approx. 35 to 40 minutes).
13. Puree with a bender to your preferred consistency (optional). Serve immediately.

Bouillabaisse

Allergies: SF, GF, DF, EF, NF

Ingredients -

- [ ] 1 pound of 3 different kinds of fish fillets
- [ ] 1/4 cup Coconut oil
- [ ] 1 pound of Oysters, clams, or mussels
- [ ] 1/3 cup cooked shrimp, crab, or lobster meat, or rock lobster tails
- [ ] 1/3 cup thinly sliced onions
- [ ] 1 Shallot or the white parts of 1 leek, thinly sliced
- [ ] 1 clove garlic, crushed
- [ ] 1 small tomato, chopped
- [ ] 1/2 sweet red pepper, chopped
- [ ] 2 stalks celery, thinly sliced
- [ ] 1-inch slice of fennel or 1/2 tsp. of fennel seed
- [ ] 1 sprigs fresh thyme or 1/4 tsp. dried thyme
- [ ] 1 bay leaf
- [ ] 1 whole cloves
- [ ] Zest of half an orange
- [ ] 1/4 tsp. saffron
- [ ] 1 teaspoons salt
- [ ] 1/4 tsp. ground black pepper
- [ ] 1/3 cup clam juice or fish broth
- [ ] 1 Tbps lemon juice
- [ ] 1/3 cup white wine

Instructions

- ☐ In a large saucepan, heat 1/8 cup of the coconut oil.
- ☐ When it is hot, add onions and shallots (or leeks). Sauté for a minute.
- ☐ Add crushed garlic and sweet red pepper.
- ☐ Add celery, tomato, and fennel.
- ☐ Stir the vegetables until well coated.
- ☐ Add another 1/8 cup of coconut oil, bay leaf, thyme, cloves, and the orange zest.
- ☐ Cook until the onion is golden.
- ☐ Cut fish fillets into 2-inch pieces.
- ☐ Add 1 cup of water and the pieces of fish to the vegetable mixture.
- ☐ Bring to a boil, reduce heat, and let it simmer, uncovered, for about 10 minutes.
- ☐ Add clams, oysters, or mussels (optional) and crabmeat, shrimp, or lobster tails, cut into pieces.
- ☐ Add salt, saffron, and pepper.
- ☐ Add lemon juice, clam juice, and white wine.
- ☐ Bring to a simmer again and cook for 5 minutes longer.

Gaspacho

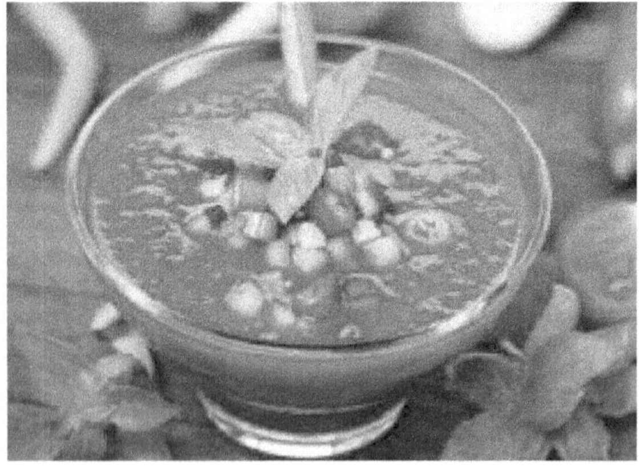

Allergies: SF, GF, DF, EF, V, NF

Ingredients –

- o 1/4 cup of flax seeds meal

- o 1 pound tomatoes, diced
- o 1 red pepper or one green pepper, diced
- o 1 small cucumber, peeled and diced
- o 1 cloves of garlic, peeled and crushed
- o ¼ cup extra virgin olive oil or cumin oil
- o 1 tbsp. lemon juice
- o Salt, to taste

Instructions

10. Mix the peppers, tomatoes, and cucumber with the crushed garlic and olive oil in a blender bowl. Add flax meal to the mixture.
11. Blend until smooth.
12. Add salt and lemon juice to taste and stir well.
13. Refrigerate. Serve with black olives, hardboiled egg, cilantro, mint or parsley.

Italian Beef Soup

Allergies: SF, GF, DF, EF, NF

Ingredients -

a. 1/3 pound minced beef
b. 1 clove garlic, minced
c. 1 cups beef broth
d. 1 large tomato
e. 1/2 cup sliced carrots
f. 1/2 cup cooked beans
g. 1 small zucchini, cubed
h. 1 cups Spinach - rinsed and torn
i. 1/8 tsp. black pepper

j.   1/8 tsp. Salt Brown Beef with Garlic in a stockpot.

- ☐ Stir in broth, carrots, and tomatoes.
- ☐ Season with salt and pepper.
- ☐ Reduce heat, cover, and simmer for 15 minutes.
- ☐ Stir in beans with li☐uid and zucchini. Cover, and simmer until zucchini is tender.
- ☐ Remove from heat, add Spinach, and cover.
- ☐ Serve after 5 minutes.

Black Bean Soup

Allergies: SF, GF, DF, EF, NF

Ingredients -

- o 1 Tbsp. cup Coconut Oil
- o 1/4 cup Onion, Diced
- o 1/4 cup Carrots, Diced
- o 1/4 cup Green Bell Pepper, Diced
- o 1 cup beef broth
- o 1 pound cooked Black Beans
- o 1 tbsp. lemon juice
- o 1 teaspoons chopped garlic
- o 1 teaspoons Salt
- o 1/4 tsp. Black Pepper, Ground
- o 1 teaspoons Chili Powder
- o 4 oz. pork
- o 1 tbsp. tapioca flour
- o 2 tbsp. Water

Instructions

- ☐ Place coconut oil, onion, carrot, and bell pepper in a stockpot.
- ☐ Cook the veggies until tender.
- ☐ Bring broth to a boil.
- ☐ Add cooked beans, broth, and the remaining ingredients (except tapioca flour and 2 tbsp. water) to the vegetables.
- ☐ Bring that mixture to a simmer and cook for approximately 15 minutes.
- ☐ Puree 1 ☐uart of the soup in a blender and put back into the pot.
- ☐ Combine the tapioca flour and 2 tbsp. Water in a separate bowl.
- ☐ Add the tapioca flour mixture to the bean soup and bring to a boil for 1 minute.

GRILLED MEATS & SALAD

Chicken and Large Fiber Loaded Salad with Italian Dressing

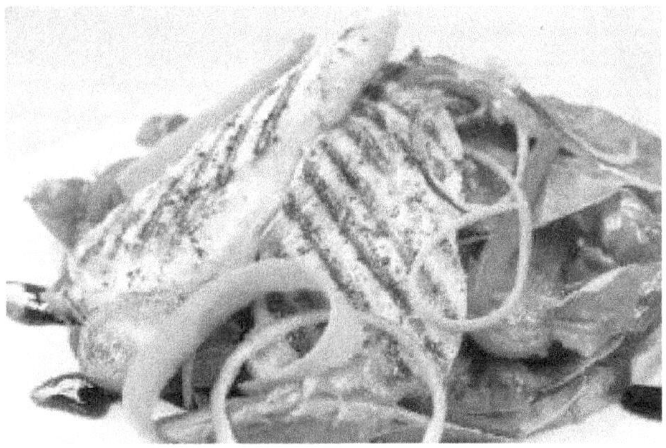

Allergies: SF, GF, EF, NF

- o   2 6oz. pieces of ChickenChicken (or turkey), skinless, boneless grilled, or prepared in the skillet.
- o   Large mixed Spinach and lettuce salad with Italian Dressing and half a tsp of mustard. Salad can be as large as you want, but use half a cup of the Dressing.

Salmon with Large Fiber Loaded Salad with Italian Dressing

Allergies: SF, GF, DF, EF, NF

5. 2 Salmon steaks grilled or prepared in the skillet.
6. Large mixed Spinach and lettuce salad with "Italian Dressing" and some thyme sprinkled on top of it. Salad can be as large as you want, but use the prescribed amount of the Dressing.

Ground Beef Patty with Large Fiber Loaded Salad with Yogurt Dressing

Allergies: SF, GF, EF, NF

5. 2 5oz. Lean ground beef patty grilled or prepared in the skillet.

6. Large mixed Spinach and shredded cabbage salad with Yogurt Dressing. Salad can be as large as you want, but use half a cup of a dressing

STEWS, CHILIES, AND CURRIES

Vegetarian Chili

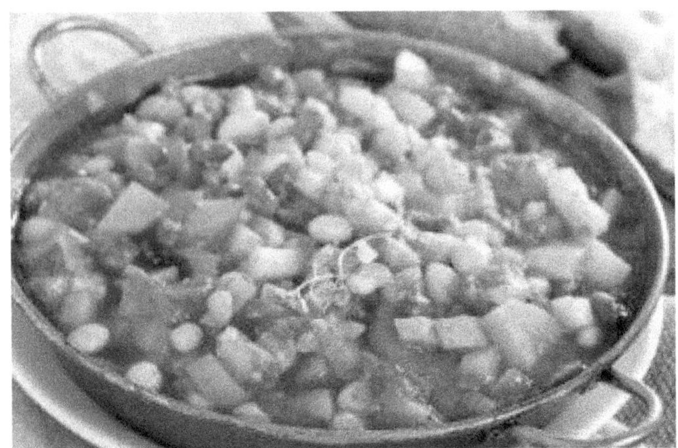

Allergies: SF, GF, DF, EF, V, NF

Ingredients -

- [ ] 1 tbsp. coconut oil
- [ ] 1/2 cup chopped onions
- [ ] 1/2 cup chopped carrots
- [ ] 1 cloves garlic, minced
- [ ] 1/2 cup chopped green bell pepper
- [ ] 1/2 cup chopped red bell pepper
- [ ] 1/4 cup chopped celery
- [ ] 1/2 tbsp. chili powder
- [ ] 1/2 cups chopped mushrooms
- [ ] 1 cup chopped tomatoes
- [ ] 1 cups cooked kidney beans
- [ ] 1/2 tbsp. ground cumin
- [ ] 1/2 teaspoons oregano
- [ ] 1/2 teaspoons crushed basil leaves

Instructions

5. Heat coconut oil in a large saucepan and add onions, carrots, and garlic; sauté until tender.

6. Stir in green pepper, red pepper, celery, and chili powder.

7. Cook, often stirring, until vegetables are tender, about 6 minutes.

8. To the vegetables, add mushrooms; cook 4 minutes. Stir in tomatoes, kidney beans, corn, cumin, oregano, and basil.

9. Bring to a boil.

10. Reduce heat to medium. Cover and simmer for 20 minutes, stirring occasionally.

Braised Green Peas with Beef

Allergies: SF, GF, DF, EF, NF

Ingredients -

- 2 cups fresh or frozen green peas
- 1 onion, finely chopped
- 2 cloves of garlic, thinly sliced and 1/2 inch of peeled/sliced fresh ginger (if you like)
- 1/2 tsp. red pepper flakes, or to taste
- 1 tomato, roughly chopped
- 2 chopped carrots
- 2 tbsp. coconut oil
- 1 cup chicken broth
- 10 oz. cubed Beef
- Salt and freshly ground black pepper

- Heat the coconut oil in a skillet over medium heat. Sauté the onion, garlic, and ginger until they are soft
- . Add the red pepper, carrot, and tomatoes and sauté until the tomato begins to soften.
- Add in the green peas.
- Add cubed Lean Beef.

□   Add in the broth and simmer over medium heat. Cover and cook until the peas are tender.

□   Season to taste with salt and pepper.

White Chicken Chili

Allergies: SF, GF, DF, EF, NF

Ingredients -

- o   2 large boneless, skinless chicken breasts
- o   1 green bell peppers
- o   1/2 yellow onion
- o   1/2 jalapeno
- o   1/4 cup diced green chilies (optional)
- o   1/4 cup of spring onions
- o   1 tbsp. coconut oil
- o   1/2 cup cooked white beans
- o   2 cups chicken or vegetable broth
- o   1/2 tsp. ground cumin
- o   1/8 tsp. cayenne pepper
- o   salt to taste

Instructions

6. Bring a pot of water to boil.
7. Add the chicken breasts and cook until cooked through.
8. Drain water and allow ChickenChicken to cool. When cold, shred and set aside.
9. Dice the bell peppers, jalapeno, and onion.
10. Melt the coconut oil in a pot over high heat.
11. Add the peppers and onions and sauté until soft, approx. 8-10 minutes.
12. Add the broth, beans, ChickenChicken, and spices to the pot.
13. Stir and bring to a low boil. Cover and simmer for 25-30 minutes.
14. Simmer for 10 more minutes and stir occasionally. Remove from heat.
15. Let stand for 10 minutes to thicken. Top with cilantro.

Kale Pork

Allergies: SF, GF, DF, EF, NF

Ingredients –

a. 1 tbsp. coconut oil
b. 1/2 pound pork tenderloin, trimmed and cut into 1-inch pieces • 1/4 tsp. salt
c. 1/2 medium onion, finely chopped
d. 2 cloves garlic, minced
e. 1 teaspoons paprika
f. 1/8 tsp. crushed red pepper (optional) • 1/2 cup white wine
g. 2 plump tomatoes, chopped
h. 2 cups chicken broth
i. 1/2 bunch kale, chopped
j. 1 cups cooked white beans

Instructions

- ☐ Heat oil in a pot over medium heat.
- ☐ Add pork, season with salt, and cook until no longer pink.
- ☐ Transfer to a plate and leave juices in the pot.
- ☐ Add onion to the pot and cook until it turns translucent
- ☐ . Add paprika, garlic, and crushed red pepper and cook for about 30 seconds.
- ☐ Add tomatoes and wine, increase heat and stir to scrape up any browned bits.
- ☐ Add broth. Bring to a boil.
- ☐ Add KaleKale and stir until it wilts.
- ☐ Lower the heat and simmer until the KaleKale is tender.
- ☐ Stir in beans, pork, and pork juices.
- ☐ Simmer for 2 more minutes.

STIR-FRIES

Pork and Bok Choy / Celery Stir Fry

Allergies: SF, GF, DF, EF, NF

10 oz. Lean Pork Tenderloin and 2 cups Bok Choy / Celery stir fry.

- ☐ Use as many veggies as you want, or replace Bok Choy with Kale. Season with fish sauce.

Lemon Chicken Stir Fry

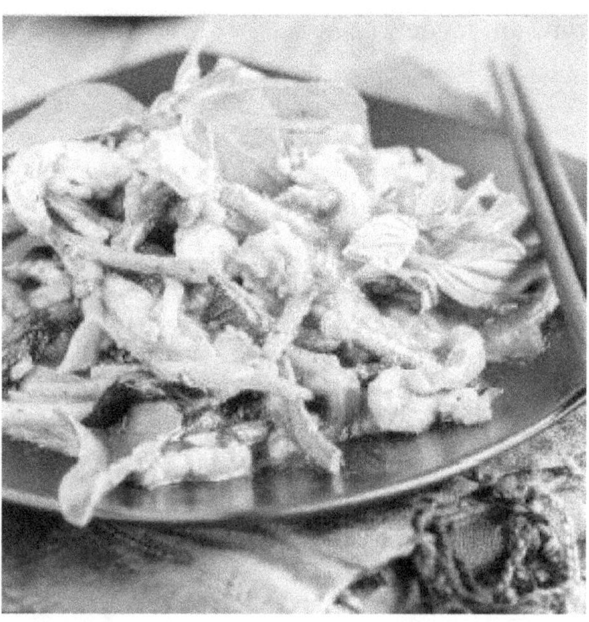

Allergies: SF, GF, DF, EF, NF

Ingredients -

- o 1/2 lemon
- o 1/4 cup chicken broth
- o 1 tbsp. fish sauce
- o 1 teaspoons arrowroot flour
- o 1/2 tbsp. coconut oil
- o 1/2 pound boneless, skinless chicken breasts, trimmed and cut into 1-inch pieces
- o 5 ounces mushrooms, halved or quartered
- o 1 cup snow peas, stems and strings removed
- o 1 bunch scallions, cut into 1-inch pieces, white and green parts divided
- o 1 tbsp. chopped garlic

Instructions

- ☐ Grate 1 tsp. Lemon zest. Juice the lemon and mix 3 tbsp. Of the juice with broth, fish sauce, and arrowroot flour in a small bowl.
- ☐ Heat oil in a skillet over high heat.
- ☐ Add ChickenChicken and cook, occasionally stirring, until just cooked through.
- ☐ Transfer to a plate.

☐ Add mushrooms to the pan and cook until the mushrooms are tender.

☐ Add snow peas, garlic, scallion whites, and the lemon zest.

☐ Cook, stirring, around 30 seconds.

☐ Add the broth to the pan and cook, stirring, 2 to 3 minutes.

☐ Add scallion greens and the ChickenChicken and any accumulated juices and stir.

Pan-seared Brussels sprouts

Serves 2

Allergies: SF, GF, DF, EF, NF

Ingredients -

    a. 6 oz. cubed pork

    b. 2 tbsp. coconut oil

    c. 1 pound Brussels sprouts, halved

    d. 1/2 large onion, chopped

    e. Salt and ground black pepper

Instructions

4. Cook pork in a skillet over high heat.
5. Remove to a plate and chop.
6. In the same pan with pork fat, add coconut oil over high heat.
7. Add onions and Brussels sprouts and cook, occasionally stirring, until sprouts are golden brown.
8. Season with salt and pepper to taste, and put the pork back into the pan.
9. Serve immediately

Beef and Broccoli Stir Fry

Allergies: SF, GF, DF, EF, NF

- 10 oz. of lean Beef and 2 cups broccoli stir fry.

- Use as much Broccoli as you want or replace Broccoli with Kale.

MEATS

Baked Chicken Breast with Fresh Basil

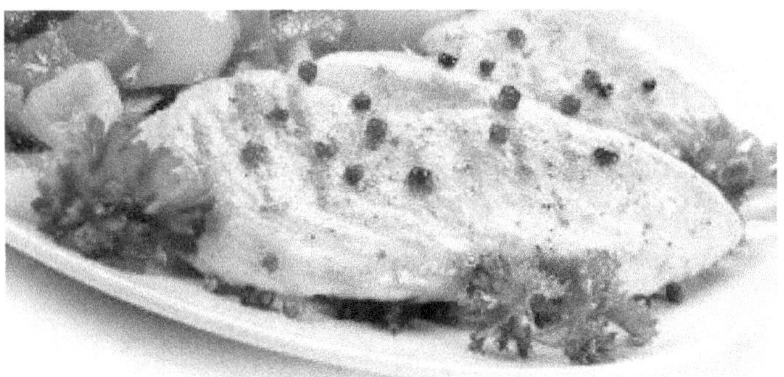

Allergies: SF, GF, EF, NF

Ingredients -

- o 2 boneless skinless chicken breast
- o 1/4 cup low-fat Yogurt
- o 1/4 cup chopped basil
- o 1 tsp. arrowroot flour
- o 2 Tbsp. oatmeal, coarsely ground

Instructions

4. Arrange ChickenChicken in a baking dish. Combine basil, Yogurt, and arrowroot flour;
5. mix well and spread over ChickenChicken.
6. Mix oatmeal with salt and pepper to taste and sprinkle over ChickenChicken.
7. Bake chicken at 375 degrees in the oven for half an hour.

Roast Chicken with Rosemary

Allergies: SF, GF, DF, EF, NF

- o 2 chicken pieces, skinned
- o salt and pepper to taste
- o 1 onion, ☐uartered
- o 2 Tbsp. chopped rosemary

Instructions -

4. Heat the oven to 350F.
5. Sprinkle meat with salt and pepper.
6. Cover with the onion and rosemary.
7. Place in a baking dish and bake in the preheated oven until ChickenChicken is cooked through.

Carne Asada

Allergies: SF, GF, DF, EF, NF

Marinade:

4. Mix the garlic, jalapeno, cilantro, salt, and pepper to make a paste.
5. Put the paste in a container.
6. Add the oil and lime juice.
7. Shake it up to combine.
8. Use as a marinade for Beef or as a table condiment.

Instructions

- [ ] Put the 1 pound flank steak in a baking dish and pour the marinade over it.
- [ ] Refrigerate up to 8 hours.
- [ ] Take the steak out of the marinade and season it on both sides with salt and pepper.
- [ ] Grill (or broil) the steak for 7 to 10 minutes per side, turning once, until medium-rare.
- [ ] Put the steak on a cutting board and allow the juices to settle (5 minutes).
- [ ] Thinly slice the steak across the grain.

CASSEROLES

Broccoli Chicken Casserole

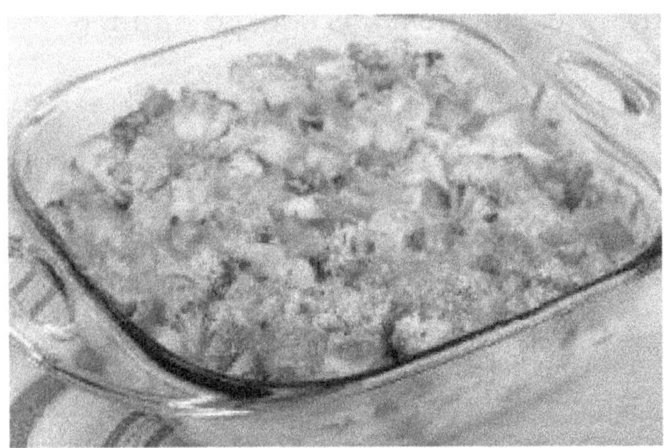

Allergies: SF, GF, NF

Ingredients -

    a. 2 cups broccoli florets

    b. 10 oz. skinless, boneless chicken (or turkey) pieces (breast or dark meat)

    c. 2 tsp of flax seeds meal

    d. Salt, pepper

    e. 2 eggs - beaten

    f. 1 cup of Yogurt Dressing (or coconut milk, if you don't like the sourish tang)

    g. 1/2 cup of chicken broth

    h. 4 tbsp. Of grated low-fat cheddar cheese,

- ☐ Heat the oven to 400°. Cook broccoli for around 5 minutes.
- ☐ Take Broccoli out and add ChickenChicken (or turkey) and simmer for 15 minutes.
- ☐ Cut ChickenChicken (or turkey) into cubes and add it to the Broccoli.
- ☐ Combine broth, flax, salt, and pepper in a pan and mix.
- ☐ Bring to a boil over high heat and cook for 1 minute, stirring constantly. Remove from heat.
- ☐ Add yogurt dressing, beaten egg, and then half of the cheese, stirring until well combined.

☐ Add sauce to broccoli mixture, and stir gently until combined.

☐ Put the mixture in a small casserole dish oiled with some coconut oil.

☐ Put remaining cheese on top, sprinkle.

☐ Bake at 400° for 50 minutes or until mixture bubbles at the edges and cheese begins to brown.

☐ Remove from oven and let cool for 5 minutes.

Beef Meatballs Broccoli Casserole

Allergies: SF, GF

Ingredients -

a. 2 cups broccoli florets

b. 10 oz. beef meatballs (see separate recipe)

c. 2 tsp of almond flour

d. Salt, pepper

e. 2 eggs - beaten

f. 1 cup of Yogurt Dressing

g. 1/2 cup of chicken broth

h. 2 tbsp. of grated low-fat cheddar cheese

Instructions

3. Heat oven to 400F. Cook broccoli for around 5 minutes.

4. Prepare beef meatballs as in the recipe above.

5. Combine broth, flour, salt, and pepper in a saucepan, stirring with a whisk until smooth.

6. Bring to a boil over medium-high heat; cook 1 minute, stirring constantly.

7. Remove from heat.

8. Add yogurt dressing, beaten egg, and then half of the cheese, stirring until well combined.

9. Add sauce to broccoli mixture, and stir gently until combined.

10. Put the mixture in a small casserole dish oiled with some coconut oil.

11. Sprinkle with remaining cheese.

12. Bake at 400° for 50 minutes or until mixture bubbles at the edges and cheese begins to brown.

13. Remove from oven and let cool for 5 minutes.

14. Serve with large Fiber Loaded Salad with Italian Dressing.

Beef Meatballs Cauliflower Casserole

Allergies: SF, GF

Ingredients -

- o 2 cups cauliflower florets
- o 10 oz. beef meatballs (see separate recipe)
- o 2 tsp of almond flour
- o Salt, pepper
- o 2 eggs - beaten
- o 1 cup of Yogurt Dressing
- o 1/2 cup of chicken broth
- o 2 tbsp of grated low-fat cheddar cheese

Instructions

- ☐ Heat oven to 400°.
- ☐ Cook cauliflower for around 5 minutes.
- ☐ Prepare beef meatballs as in the recipe above. Combine soup, flour, salt, and pepper in a saucepan, stirring with a whisk until smooth. Bring to a boil over medium-high heat; cook 1 minute, stirring constantly.
- ☐ Remove from heat.
- ☐ Add yogurt dressing, beaten egg, and then half of the cheese, stirring until well combined.

☐ Add sauce to the cauliflower mixture, and stir gently until combined.

☐ Put the mixture in a small casserole dish oiled with some coconut oil. Sprinkle with remaining cheese.

☐ Bake at 400° for 50 minutes or until mixture bubbles at the edges and cheese begins to brown. Remove from oven and let cool for 5 minutes.

☐ Serve with large Fiber Loaded Salad with Italian Dressing.

"BREADED" "FRIED" FOOD

Breaded Tilapia

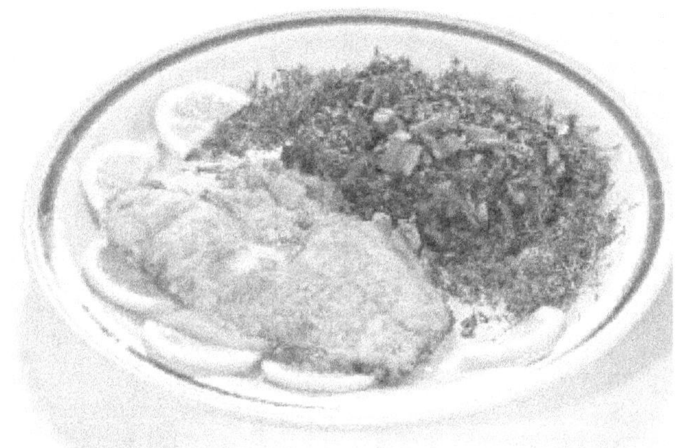

Allergies: SF, GF, DF, NF

Ingredients -

- o 1/2 cup coconut meal for breading
- o 1/4 tsp. pepper
- o 1/4 tsp. minced garlic
- o 1/4 tsp. paprika
- o 1/8 tsp. salt
- o 1 large egg whites (or whole eggs), beaten
- o 1/2 pound tilapia fillets, cut into 1/2-by-3-inch strips

Instructions

- ☐ Heat oven to 400°F. Set a wire rack on a baking sheet and coat with some coconut oil.
- ☐ Place coconut, pepper, Garlic, paprika, and salt in a blender and process until finely.
- ☐ Transfer to a shallow dish.
- ☐ Place egg whites in a second dish. Dip every piece of fish in the egg and then coat all sides with the coconut breading mixture.
- ☐ Place on the prepared rack.
- ☐ Sprinkle some drops of olive oil over each piece.
- ☐ Bake until the fish is cooked through. Breading should be golden brown.
- ☐ Serve with large FiberFiber loaded salad.

Breaded Chicken

Allergies: SF, GF, DF, NF

Ingredients -

- o 1/2 cup flax seeds meal for breading
- o 1/4 tsp. pepper
- o 1/4 tsp. minced garlic
- o 1/4 tsp. paprika
- o 1/8 tsp. salt
- o 1 large egg whites (or whole eggs), beaten
- o 1/2 pound skinless, boneless chicken pieces

Instructions

4. Heat oven to 400°F. Set a wire rack on a baking sheet; coat with some coconut oil.
5. Place flax, pepper, Garlic, paprika, and salt in a food processor or blender and process until finely.
6. Transfer to a shallow dish.

7. Place egg whites in a second dish. Dip every piece of ChickenChicken in the egg and then coat all sides with the flax breading mixture.

8. Place on the prepared rack.

9. Sprinkle some drops of olive oil over each piece.

10. Bake until the ChickenChicken is cooked through, and the breading is golden brown and crisp, about 8 minutes each side.

11. Serve with a large FiberFiber loaded salad.

Lemon Pork with Asparagus

Allergies: SF, GF, DF, EF, NF

Ingredients -

- o 1/2 lb. pork chops
- o 2 Tbsp. buckwheat flour
- o 1/4 tsp. salt
- o 1 tbsp. coconut oil
- o Pepper
- o 1/2 cup chopped asparagus
- o 1 lemons, sliced

Instructions

- ☐ Place the flour and salt in a dish and gently toss each chop in the dish to coat. Melt the coconut oil in a large skillet over medium-high heat.
- ☐ Add the ChickenChicken and sauté until golden brown on each side.
- ☐ Sprinkle each side with the pepper directly in the pan.
- ☐ When the chops are cooked through, transfer them to a plate.
- ☐ Add the lemon slices and asparagus to the pan.
- ☐ When the asparagus and the lemons are done, add the chops back to the pan.

PIZZA

Meat Pizza

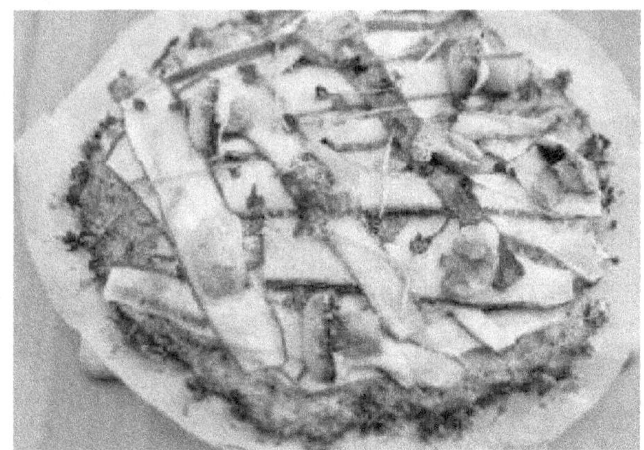

Allergies: SF, GF, EF, NF

Ingredients -

- o 1/2 cup cooked and minced chicken breast
- o 1/2 cup low-fat cheddar, shredded
- o 1/2 tbsp. minced onion & few basil leaves
- o 1/2 tsp garlic minced

Instructions

6. Preheat oven to 425 degrees Fahrenheit. Process chicken, onion, and garlic together.

7. The mixture will be a dense crumb consistency.

8. Press chicken mixture on parchment paper on a cookie sheet. Bake for 12 minutes. Let cool for five minutes.

9. Top with 1/4 cup of tomato sauce, a handful of low-fat cheese, basil, and mushrooms (shiitake). Bake for 6-8 minutes more, or until toppings are melted.

10. Let cool for five minutes. Slice and serve. Alternatively, you may want to try the cauliflower crust version:

11. Grate half of the large Cauliflower and steam it for 15 minutes.

12. Squeeze the excess water out and let cool. Mix in 2 eggs, one cup low-fat mozzarella, and salt and pepper.

13. Pat into a 10-inch round on the prepared cookie sheet.

14. Brush with oil and bake until golden. Add the topping as above.

SIDE DISHES

Roasted curried Cauliflower

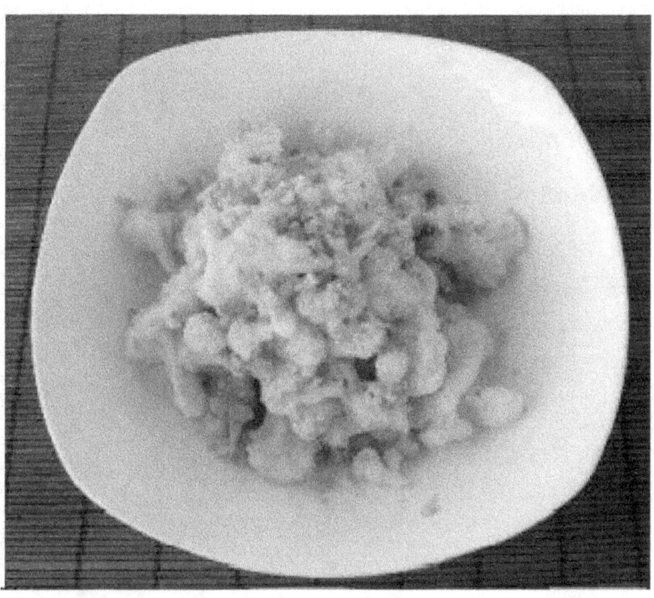

Allergies: SF, GF, DF, EF, NF

Ingredients -

- o 2 cups cauliflower florets
- o 1/2 chopped small onion
- o 1/4 tsp. coriander seeds
- o 1/4 tsp. cumin seeds
- o 2 Tbsp. cup olive oil or cumin oil
- o 1/4 cup lemon juice
- o 1 teaspoon curry paste
- o 1/4 tbsp. hot paprika
- o 1/4 teaspoons salt
- o 2 tbsp. cup chopped cilantro

Instructions

7. Heat oven to 450°F. Place cauliflower florets in a large roasting pan.
8. Add onions to Cauliflower.
9. Dry toast coriander and cumin seeds in a skillet over medium heat until slightly browned, about 5 minutes.
10. Crush in a mortar with pestle.

11. Place seeds in a bowl. Whisk in oil, lemon juice, curry paste, paprika, and salt.

12. Pour Dressing over vegetables and toss to coat.

13. Spread vegetables in a single layer and sprinkle with pepper.

14. Roast vegetables until tender, occasionally stirring, about 35 minutes.

15. Sprinkle cilantro and serve warm.

Roasted Cauliflower with Tahini sauce

Allergies: SF, GF, DF, EF, V, NF

Ingredients -

- o 2 Tbsp. cup extra-virgin olive oil or avocado oil

- o 1 tsp. ground cumin

- o 1 smaller cauliflower head, cored and cut into 1 1/2" florets

- o Salt and ground black pepper

- o 1/4 cup tahini

- o 1 cloves garlic, smashed and minced into a paste

- o Juice of 1/4 lemon

Instructions

4. Roast Cauliflower like in the previous recipe.
5. Meanwhile, combine tahini, lemon juice, garlic, and 1/4 cup water in a bowl and season with salt.
   Serve Cauliflower hot or at room temperature with tahini sauce.

Asparagus with mushrooms and hazelnuts

Ingredients - Allergies: SF, GF, DF, EF, V

- o   1 tbsp. lemon juice
- o   1/8 tsp sea salt
- o   Ground black pepper, to taste
- o   1/2 pound fresh asparagus, ends trimmed
- o   1 tbsp. coconut oil
- o   2 cups mushrooms
- o   1/4 cup green onions, sliced
- o   1 tbsp. hazelnuts, toasted and finely chopped

Instructions

- ☐   Add the lemon juice, 1/2 tbsp. Of the oil, salt, and pepper in a small bowl
- ☐   . Boil water in a pan and add the asparagus.
- ☐   Boil for few minutes.
- ☐   Heat the remaining 1/2 tbsp.
- ☐   Oil in a pan on high heat.
- ☐   Add mushrooms and cook them until they are soft.
- ☐   Add green onions and sauté one more minute.
- ☐   Add the asparagus, and cook for another 3 minutes.
- ☐   Remove from the heat and slowly add in the lemon juice mixture.
- ☐   Add the toasted hazelnuts over the top.

Chard and Cashew Sauté

Serves 2

Allergies: SF, GF, DF, EF, V, NF

Ingredients -

- o 1 bunch Swiss chard
- o 1/2 cup cashews
- o 1 tbsp. coconut oil
- o Sea salt (optional)
- o ground black pepper

Instructions

- ☐ Wash Swiss chard and remove tough stems.
- ☐ Heat a skillet over medium heat, and add oil when hot.
- ☐ Chop Swiss chard into thin strips.
- ☐ Add Swiss chard to the hot skillet, along with cashews.
- ☐ Sauté only 1 minute.
- ☐ Season with sea salt and ground black pepper to taste and serve warm.

Cauliflower rice side dish

Serves 2

Allergies: SF, GF, DF, EF, V, NF

Ingredients -

- o 1 head Cauliflower
- o 2 Tbs coconut oil
- o Sea salt, garlic, ginger, or ground black pepper (optional seasonings)

Instructions

17. Place the cauliflower into a food processor and pulse it until a grainy rice-like consistency.
18. Season with sea salt and ground black pepper.
19. Meanwhile, heat a large pan over medium heat.
20. Add coconut oil when hot.

21. Sauté Cauliflower in a pan with oil and any additional seasonings if desired.

CROCKPOT

Slow Cooker Pepper Steak

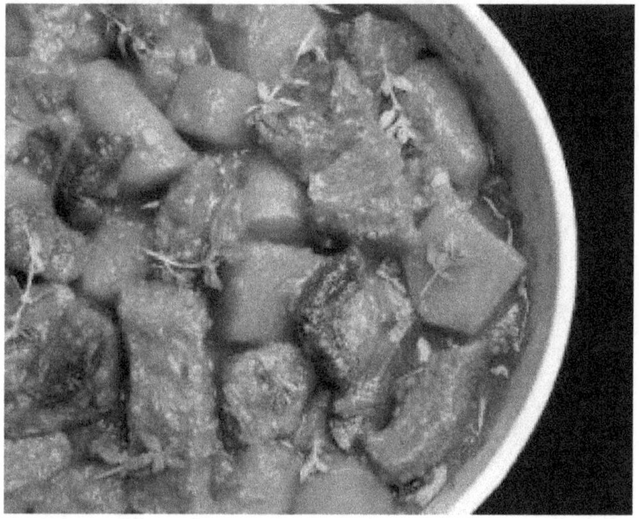

Allergies: SF, GF, DF, EF, NF

Ingredients -

- o 1 pounds beef sirloin, cut into 2-inch strips
- o 1/2 tbsp. minced garlic
- o 1 tbsp. coconut oil
- o 1/2 cup Beef Broth
- o 1/2 tbsp. tapioca flour
- o 1/4 cup chopped onion
- o 1 cup carrots

- o 1/2 cup chopped tomatoes
- o 1/2 tsp. salt

Instructions

- ☐ Sprinkle Beef with Minced Garlic.
- ☐ Heat the coconut oil in a skillet and brown the seasoned beef sirloin strips.
- ☐ Transfer to a slow cooker.
- ☐ Mix in tapioca flour in broth until dissolved.
- ☐ Pour broth into the slow cooker with meat.
- ☐ Add carrots, onion, chopped tomatoes, and salt.
- ☐ Cover and cook on high for 3 to 4 hours, or on Low for 6 to 8 hours.

Pork Tenderloin with peppers and onions

Allergies: SF, GF, DF, EF, NF

Ingredients -

- o 1 tbsp. coconut oil
- o 3/4 pound pork loin
- o 1/2 tbsp. caraway seeds
- o 1/4 tsp sea salt
- o 1/8 tsp ground black pepper
- o 1/2 red onion, thinly sliced
- o 1 red bell peppers, sliced
- o 2 cloves of garlic, minced
- o 1/4 cup chicken broth

Instructions

- ☐ Wash and chop vegetables. Slice pork loin, and season with black pepper, caraway seeds, and sea salt.

- ☐ Heat a pan over medium heat.
- ☐ Add coconut oil when hot.
- ☐ Add pork loin and brown slightly.
- ☐ Add onions and mushrooms, and continue to sauté until onions are translucent.
- ☐ Add peppers, garlic, and chicken broth.
- ☐ Simmer until vegetables are tender and pork is fully cooked

Beef Bourguinon

Allergies: SF, GF, DF, EF

Ingredients -

    a. 3/4 or 1 pound cubed Lean Beef

    b. 1/4 cup red wine

    c. 2 Tbsp. coconut oil

    d. 1/4 tsp. thyme

    e. 1/4 tsp. black pepper

    f. 1 cloves garlic, crushed

    g. 1/2 onion, diced

    h. 1/3 pound mushrooms, sliced

    i. 2 Tbsp. cup almond flour

Instructions

7. Marinate Beef in wine, oil, thyme, and pepper for a few hours at room temperature or 6-8 hours in the fridge.
8. Cook garlic and onion in a pan until soft.

9. Add mushrooms.

10. Cook until they are browned.

11. Drain beef li□uid.

12. Place Beef in the slow cooker.

13. Sprinkle flour over the beef and stir to coat.

14. Add the mushroom mixture on top.

15. Pour reserved marinade over all. Cook on low for 7-9 hrs.

Italian Chicken

Allergies: SF, GF, DF, EF

Ingredients -

- 2 pieces of skinless ChickenChicken
- 2 Tbsp. almond flour
- 1/2 tsp. salt
- 1/8 tsp. pepper
- 1/4 cup chicken broth
- 1/2 cup sliced mushrooms
- 1/4 tsp. paprika
- 1/2 zucchini, sliced into medium pieces
- ground black pepper
- parsley to garnish

Instructions

- Season chicken with 1 tsp. Salt.
- Combine flour, pepper, remaining salt, and paprika. Coat chicken pieces with this mixture.
- Place zucchini first in a crockpot.
- Pour broth over zucchini.

☐ Arrange ChickenChicken on top.

☐ Cover and cook on Low for 6 to 8 hours or until tender.

☐ Turn control to high, add mushrooms, cover, and cook on high for additional 10-15 minutes.

☐ Garnish with parsley and ground black pepper.

Slow Cook Jambalaya

Allergies: SF, GF, DF, EF, NF

Ingredients -

    a. 1/2 Bell pepper, chopped

    b. 1/2 Onion, chopped

    c. 1 Medium tomato, chopped

    d. 1/2 cup Chopped celery

    e. 1 Clove garlic, crushed

    f. 1 tbsp. minced parsley

    g. 1 tbsp. Chopped thyme leaves

    h. 1 tbsp. chopped oregano leaves

    i. 1/8 tsp. Cayenne & 1/4 tsp. Salt

    j. 4 ounces pork, chopped

    k. 4 ounces Chicken breast, chopped

    l. 1 cups Beef broth

    m. 1/4 pound Cooked shelled shrimp

    n. 1/4 cup Cooked brown rice

Instructions

☐ Shell shrimp and halve lengthwise.

☐ Combine all ingredients except shrimp & rice in a slow cooker.

☐ Cover & cook on low 9-10 hours.

- ☐ Turn slow cooker on high, add cooked shrimp & cooked rice.
- ☐ Cover; cook on high 20-30 minutes.

Ropa Vieja

Allergies: SF, GF, DF, EF, NF

Ingredients -

- o 1 tbsp. coconut oil
- o 3/4 or 1 pound beef flank steak
- o 1/2 cup beef broth
- o 1/2 cup tomato sauce
- o 1 small onion, sliced
- o 1/2 green bell pepper sliced into strips
- o 1 cloves garlic, chopped
- o 1/4 cup tomato paste
- o 1/2 tsp. ground cumin
- o 1/2 tsp. chopped cilantro
- o 1/2 tbsp. Olive oil or avocado oil & 1 tbsp. lemon juice

Instructions

- ☐ Heat oil in a skillet over high heat. Brown the flank steak on each side (4 minutes per side).
- ☐ Move the Beef to a slow cooker.
- ☐ Add in the beef broth and tomato sauce, then add the onion, bell pepper, garlic, tomato paste, cumin, cilantro, olive oil, and lemon juice.
- ☐ Stir until blended.
- ☐ Cover, and cook on high for 4 hours or on Low for up to 8 hours.
- ☐ When ready to serve, shred meat and serve with salad.

Lemon Roast Chicken

Allergies: SF, GF, DF, EF, NF

Ingredients -

- o 2 pieces skinless ChickenChicken
- o 1 dash Salt
- o 1 dash Pepper
- o 1 tsp. Oregano
- o 1 cloves minced garlic
- o 1 tbsp. coconut oil
- o 1/4 cup water
- o 1 tbsp. Lemon juice
- o Rosemary

Instructions

12. Wash Chicken and season with salt and pepper.
13. Sprinkle half of oregano and garlic inside the chicken cavity.
14. Add coconut oil to a frying pan.
15. Brown Chicken on all sides and transfer to crockpot.
16. Sprinkle with oregano and garlic.
17. Add water to the frying pan and stir to loosen brown bits.
18. Pour into the crockpot and cover.
19. Cook on low 7 hours.
20. Add lemon juice when cooking is done.
21. Transfer chicken to cutting board and carve ChickenChicken.
22. Skim fat. Pour the juice into the sauce bowl.
23. Serve with rosemary and some juice over ChickenChicken.

Fall Lamb and Vegetable Stew

Allergies: SF, GF, DF, EF, NF

Ingredients -

- o 3/4 or 1 pound Lamb stew meat
- o 1 chopped Tomatoes
- o 1/2 Summer s□uash
- o 1/2 Zucchini
- o 1/2 cup Mushrooms, sliced
- o 1/2 cup Bell peppers, chopped
- o 1/2 cup Onions, chopped
- o 1/2 teaspoons Salt
- o 1 Garlic cloves, crushed
- o 1/4 tsp. Thyme leaves
- o 1 Bay leaves
- o 1 cups chicken broth

Instructions

- ☐ Cut s□uash and zucchini.
- ☐ Place vegetables and lamb in the crockpot.
- ☐ Mix salt, garlic, thyme, and bay leaf into the broth and pour over lamb and vegetables.
- ☐ Cover and cook on Low for 7 hours.

FISH

Cioppino

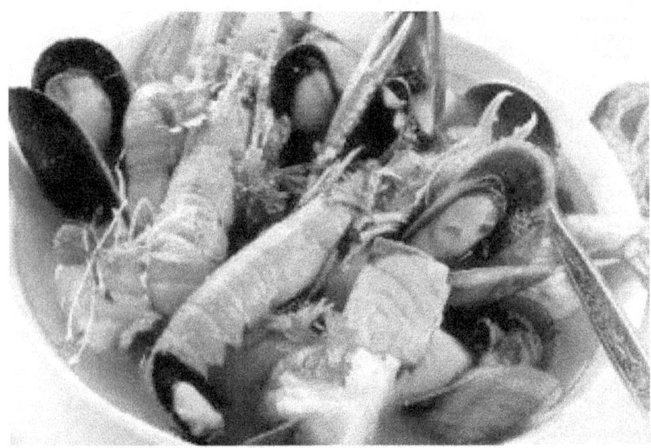

Allergies: SF, GF, DF, EF, NF

Ingredients -

- o 1/4 cup coconut oil
- o 1 onions, chopped
- o 1 cloves garlic, minced
- o 1/2 bunch fresh parsley, chopped
- o 1/2 cup stewed tomatoes
- o 1/2 cups chicken broth
- o 1 bay leaves
- o 1/2 tbsp. dried basil
- o 1/4 tsp. dried thyme
- o 1/4 tsp. dried oregano
- o 1/2 cup water
- o 1/2 cup white wine
- o 1/2 pound peeled and deveined large shrimp
- o 1/2 pound bay scallops
- o 6 small clams
- o 6 cleaned and debearded mussels
- o 1/2 cups crabmeat
- o 1/2 pounds cod fillets, cubed

Instructions

13. Over medium heat, melt coconut oil in a large stockpot and add onions, parsley, and garlic. Cook slowly, stirring occasionally until onions are soft.

14. Add tomatoes to the pot.

15. Add chicken broth, oregano, bay leaves, basil, thyme, water, and wine.

16. Mix well. Cover and simmer 30 minutes.

17. Stir in the shrimp, scallops, clams, mussels, and crabmeat.

18. Stir in fish.

19. Bring to boil. Lower heat, cover and simmer until clams open.

Flounder with Orange Coconut Oil

Allergies: SF, GF, DF, EF, NF

Ingredients -

    a. 1 pound flounder

    b. 1 tbsp. white wine

    c. 1 tbsp. lemon juice

    d. 1 tbsp. coconut oil

    e. 1 tbsp. parsley

    f. 1/3 tsp. black pepper

    g. 1 tbsp. orange zest

    h. 1/4 tsp. salt

    i. 1/4 cup chopped scallions

Instructions

☐ Preheat oven to 325F. Sprinkle fish with pepper and salt.

☐ Place fish in the baking dish. Sprinkle orange zest on top of the fish.

☐ Melt remaining coconut oil and add the parsley and scallions to the coconut oil and pour over flounder.

☐ Then add in the white wine.

☐ Place in oven and bake for 15 minutes.

☐ Serve fish with extra juice on a side.

Grilled Salmon

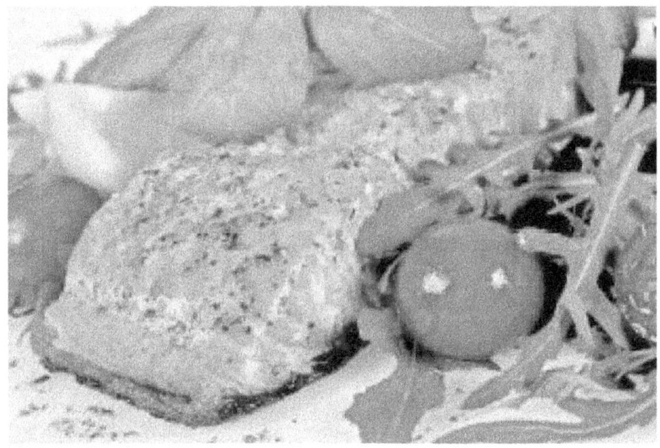

Allergies: SF, GF, DF, EF, NF

Ingredients -

- o 2 salmon filets
- o 2 Tbsp. coconut oil
- o 1 tbsp. fish sauce
- o 1 tbsp. lemon juice
- o 1 tbsp. thinly sliced green onion
- o 1 clove garlic, minced & 1/4 tsp. ground ginger
- o 1/4 tsp. crushed red pepper flakes
- o 1/4 tsp. sesame oil
- o 1/8 tsp. Salt

9. Whisk together coconut oil, fish sauce, garlic, ginger, red chili flakes, lemon juice, green onions, sesame oil, and salt.

10. Put fish in a glass dish, and pour marinade over.

11. Cover and refrigerate for 4 hours.

12. Preheat grill. Place salmon on the grill.

13. Grill until fish becomes tender.

14. Turn halfway during cooking.

Crab Cakes

Allergies: SF, GF, DF, NF

Ingredients -

- 1 lbs. crabmeat
- 1 beaten eggs
- 1 cup flax seeds meal
- 1 tbsp. mustard
- 1 tbsp. grated horseradish
- 1/4 cup coconut oil
- 1/2 tsp. lemon rind
- 1 tbsp. lemon juice
- 1 tbsp. parsley
- 1/4 tsp. cayenne pepper
- 1 tsp. fish sauce

Instructions

- In a medium bowl, combine all ingredients except oil.
- Shape into small hamburgers.

- ☐ In fry pan, heat oil and cook patties for 3-4 minutes on each side or until golden brown.
- ☐ Optionally, bake them in the oven.
- ☐ Serve as appetizers or as the main course with a large fiber salad.

SWEETS

Fruits dipped in chocolate.

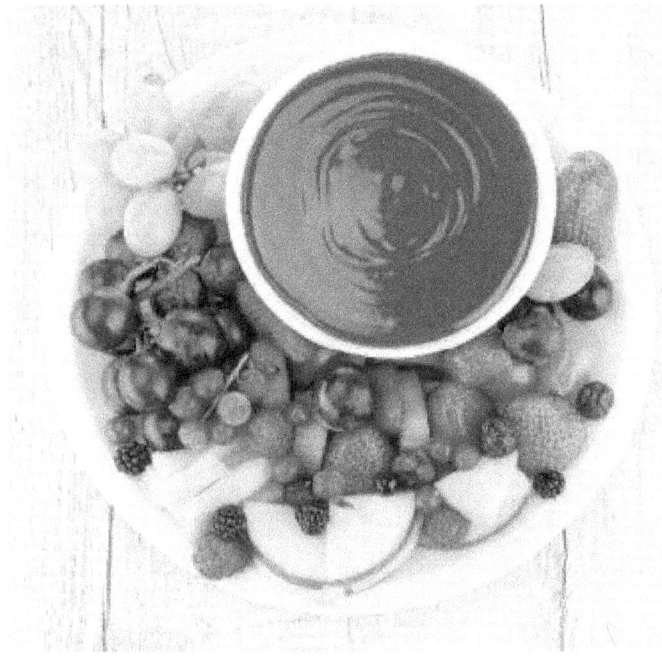

Allergies: SF, GF, DF, EF, V

Ingredients -

- o 1 apple or 1 banana or a bowl of strawberries or any fruit that can be dipped in melted chocolate
- o 1/2 cup of melted superfoods chocolate (see earlier recipe)

o   2 tbsp. chopped nuts (almond, walnut, Brazil nuts) or seeds (hemp, chia, sesame, flax meal)

Instructions

- Cut the apple in wedges or cut the banana in ▢uarters.
- Melt the chocolate and chop the nuts.
- Dip fruit in chocolate, sprinkle with nuts or seeds, and lay on the tray.
- Transfer the tray to the fridge so the chocolate can harden; serve. If you don't want chocolate, cover fruits with almond or sunflower butter and sprinkle with chia or hemp seeds and cut it into chunks and serve.

Whipped Coconut cream

Allergies: SF, GF, DF, EF, V, NF

Ingredients -

o   2 cups of any fresh berries

o   1/2 lemons

o   1 can full-fat coconut milk (14 oz.), refrigerated overnight

o   1 tsp of ground vanilla bean

o   2 Tbsp. lucuma powder

o   Dash of cardamom, nutmeg, and clove (optional)

Instructions

8. Different coconut cream from the milk by putting it overnight in the fridge.
9. Don't shake it before opening.
10. Open the can of coconut milk and scrape out the cream into a bowl.
11. Use the saved milk for smoothies or other recipes.
12. Add cardamom, lucuma powder, and vanilla.
13. Whip the cream with a hand mixer until fluffy. Put in the fridge.
14. Wash berries and place them in serving bowls or glasses.
15. S▢ueeze the lemon over the berries.
16. Place a big scoop of cream on top of the berries and serve.

Ice cream

Allergies: SF, GF, DF, EF, V, NF

Freeze a banana cut into chunks and process it in a blender once frozen and add half a tsp. of cinnamon or 1 tsp. Of cocoa or both and eat it like ice-cream.

Other option would be to add one spoon of almond butter and mix it with mashed banana, it's also a delicious ice cream

CONCLUSION

If you have diabetes, your body cannot make or properly use insulin. This leads to high blood glucose, or blood sugar, levels. Healthy eating helps keep your blood sugar in your target range. It is a critical part of managing your diabetes because controlling your blood sugar can prevent the complications of diabetes.

A registered dietitian can help make an eating plan just for you. It should take into account your weight, medicines, lifestyle, and other health problems you have.

Healthy diabetic eating includes

- Limiting foods that are high in sugar
- Eating smaller portions, spread out over the day.
- Being careful about when and how many carbohydrates you eat
- Eating a variety of whole-grain foods, fruits, and vegetables every day.
- Eating less fat
- Limiting your use of alcohol
- Using less saltv